ANTHROPOLOGICAL PAPERS

MUSEUM OF ANTHROPOLOGY, UNIVERSITY OF MICHIGAN

NO. 60

LAS YERBAS DE LA GENTE: A STUDY OF HISPANO-AMERICAN MEDICINAL PLANTS

BY
KAREN COWAN FORD

ANN ARBOR
THE UNIVERSITY OF MICHIGAN, 1975

ISBN (print): 978-0-932206-58-9
ISBN (ebook): 978-1-951519-11-7

Browse all of our books at
sites.lsa.umich.edu/archaeology-books.

Order our books from the University of Michigan
Press at www.press.umich.edu.

For permissions, questions, or manuscript queries,
contact Museum publications by email at umma-pubs@umich.edu or visit the Museum website at
lsa.umich.edu/ummaa.

ACKNOWLEDGEMENTS

My interest in Hispanic American medicinal herbs grew in part from assisting Richard I. Ford in his study of the ecology of San Juan Pueblo, a Tewa-speaking Indian group on the Rio Grande in northern New Mexico, which was funded by National Science Foundation Grant #659. In studying Pueblo Indian uses of plants it was necessary to examine Spanish-named plants and the interactions between the Pueblos and their Spanish-speaking neighbors. In the course of this research I became aware of several unpublished collections of Spanish-named plants, mostly at the University of Michigan Museum of Anthropology. The study of these collections, as well as my continuing fieldwork, has been supported by a Wenner-Gren Foundation for Anthropological Research Museum Research Fellowship (Grant #1956-1829 plus a supplemental grant). Without the Foundation's continued appreciation for this project and understanding of unexpected delays these collections would have remained unstudied.

These investigations were conducted under the guidance of Professor Volney H. Jones who gave permission to use the facilities and files of the Museum of Anthropology's Ethnobotanical Laboratory at the University of Michigan. Professor Jones, Dr. Carroll L. Riley, Dr. Anne Smith, and the late Dr. Edward P. Dozier kindly provided access to unpublished materials. Dr. Bertha Dutton, Dr. Alfonso Ortiz, Mr. and Mrs. Hugo Crowder, and many other friends and informants assisted in my fieldwork. Library and bibliographic assistance was provided by Dr. Nancie L. Gonzales and Mrs. Mary Bryan while Dr. Rogers McVaugh helped greatly with the botanical nomenclature. Miss Dorothy Kent and the late Miss Anne Avery supplied advice and encouragement and the former provided lodging in an ideal location for my fieldwork. Mr. Gary Clark assisted in the processing of the data, Mrs. Judith Hsieh, Ms. Dorothy Eckoff, Ms. Nancy Nowak, and Ms. Mary Hodge of the Museum of Anthropology of the University of Michigan as well as Ms. Lucinda Quackenbush provided secretarial services, and Mr. George Stuber contributed the map. Editing by Ms. Barbara Bluestone and Ms. Mary Coombs is greatly appreciated. Finally, my husband, Dr. Richard I. Ford, has provided constant encouragement and invaluable assistance in all phases of this project.

CAUTION !!!

The various ethnic groups included in this study have many members who know and use herbal remedies. These people know the area in which they live very well and know where their relatives and teachers collected herbs and how they used them. The use of wild plants as medicines involves little risk to these individuals, their families, and friends. Let me strongly caution others who are reading this report, however: plants of the same species growing in different areas may have different properties, with some having toxic effects; some parts of a particular species of plant may be safe to use while other parts are poisonous; some plants may be safe only at particular points in their life cycle; and, finally, it is at times quite difficult to distinguish a poisonous species from an edible one within the same plant family. Please seek the assistance of a qualified botanist to identify any wild plants before ingesting them.

TABLE OF CONTENTS

INTRODUCTION

Medicinal herb lore of Hispanic America, the area of Spanish settlement in the New World, has fascinated scholars and laymen for many years. A rich body of herb knowledge is to be found among the inhabitants of the northern part of this area. During the past 40 years a number of individuals have tapped this valuable knowledge of plants and collected data on usage, and much of this remains unpublished.

Several unpublished collections of herbs are housed in the Ethnobotanical Laboratory at the University of Michigan. These have been used in this study and will be briefly described here. In 1932 Volney H. Jones purchased a number of herbs from market vendors in Juarez, Chihuahua, Mexico. After collecting local names and information on use, he identified the specimens botanically (Appendix A). Two years later A. Whiting and C.C. Lundell obtained economic plants from markets and in the field in the Mexican states of San Luís Potosí and Nueva Leon. Usage data and Spanish names were collected and botanical identifications were made (Appendix B). Leslie A. White purchased samples of dried herbs, each labeled with a Spanish name, from a prescription druggist, B. Ruppe, in Albuquerque, New Mexico, in 1941 (Appendix C). Richard I. Ford and I purchased a portion of the inventory of an herb dealer in the Juarez market in 1965 for comparative purposes and to assist our work with Pueblo Indians in northern New Mexico. Names and uses were obtained and identifications were made (Appendix D). The Roybal's Store Collection (Appendix E), obtained by Karen Cowan Ford in 1966, includes names, information about sources, usages, and clientele, as well as botanical identifications. In addition, C. Riley and C. Trujillo (of Southern Illinois University) made available to me a manuscript (circa 1956) describing plants with names and medicinal uses from the Mexican states of Durango and Zacatecas. Finally, S. Schulman and A. Smith's research report (1962) included many Spanish-named herbs from northern New Mexico along with common English plant names and considerable usage data. All of these studies remain unpublished, but are included in my glossary (Appendix F).

The disparate nature of these studies prohibited full utilization without supplementing them with additional fieldwork in the northern part of the area, especially northern New Mexico. It has been my task to place this information in a wider social context and to assemble the data into a useful format for other scholars. In order to facilitate further study and specifically to create this format, a glossary (Appendix F) of Spanish-named medicinal herbs was compiled using the names and botanical identifications from the collections as well as several published works to add depth and geographical breadth. Particularly

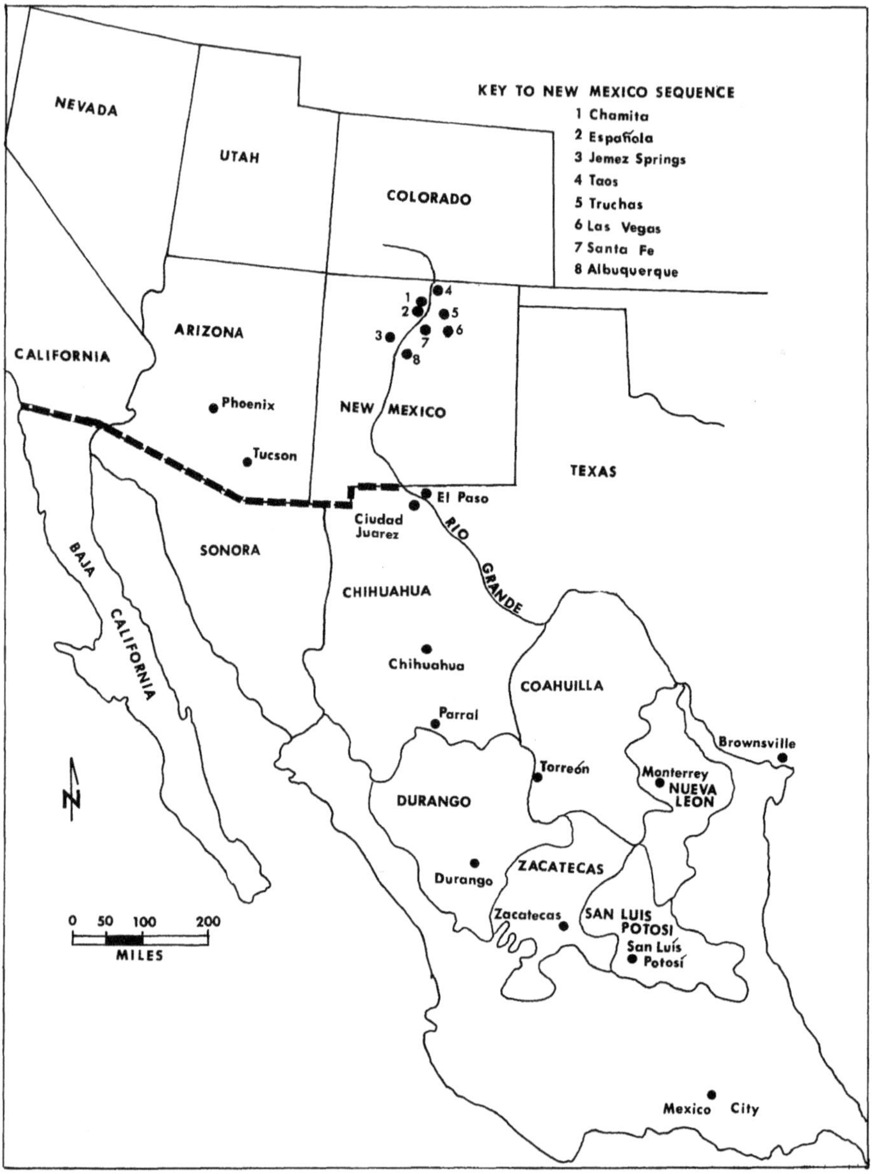

Fig. 1. Geographical area under study.

significant sources covering regions within the area under study were Kelly (1965) on Coahuilla, Zingg (1932) on Chihuahua, Owen (1963) on Baja California, Robbins et al. (1916) and Curtin (1947) on New Mexico, and Pennington (1963a, 1963b) on the Tepehuan and the Tarahumar. The following, though from outside the area of major concern, were also used: Madsen (1965), Field (1953), and Redfield (1928), all on the Valley of Mexico. As it has developed, this glossary will serve as a useful reference for others interested in medicinal herbs.*

Since this research was designed to analyze existing museum collections, these, in turn, delineated the geographical area to be considered, which extends from San Luís Potosí to Baja California to northern New Mexico and includes all or part of the Mexican states of Nueva Leon, Coahuila, San Luís Potosí, Durango, Zacatecas, Chihuahua, Sonora, and parts of the American states of Texas, New Mexico, Arizona, Colorado, and California (see Fig. 1). This area includes the Rio Grande Valley and adjacent semi-arid uplands as well as the Chihuahuan and Sonoran deserts and semi-arid uplands to the east, south, and north. Despite its extent, fortunately, this region is a manageable unit of analysis from the perspective of herbal lore. Since folk medicine is known only superficially for some of this area, emphasis of necessity will be placed on the eastern two-thirds of the region. The Sonoran Desert and environs will only be dealt with tangentially.

The culturally diverse inhabitants of this geographical area include various Indian tribes, mestizos, Hispanos (Spanish-speakers in the southwestern U.S. descended from seventeenth and eighteenth century settlers), Mexican-Americans, Chicanos, Blacks, Anglos, and commune groups. No systematic attempt has been made to study the herb lore of the various Indian tribes, but they have long intermingled with people of Spanish descent, exchanging plants and plant names; thus, groups such as the Tepehuan, Tarahumara, Pima, Keres, Tewa, and Tiwa are included in the study. Anglos in the southwestern United States have not been systematically included in my research but some, particularly those living in rural communes, have been indirectly observed, and a few brief comments will be included. For the most part the people involved with the herbs under study are Hispanos in the United States and mestizos in Mexico living in villages and urban centers. Over northern Hispanic America these people share a heritage that includes folk Catholicism and herbal curing based on certain disease concepts, despite differences in economic pursuits.

Within this area there is, however, considerable diversity of herbal knowledge, use, and procurement. Inhabitants of various areas have differential access to different plant habitats,

* The Botanical Name Dictionary (Appendix G) facilitates retrieving information about plants when the Spanish name is not known.

e.g., desert, mountains. The history of individual locales within the area has varied in the extent of interaction among different cultural groups, e.g., Indian tribes, Anglos. Availability of Western culture -- medicine, stores, and religious groups -- has been differential. In any case, since the fund of medicinal information throughout the area precludes everyone being an expert and prevents any one person from knowing all, I hypothesize an hierarchy of knowledge about the medico-health system and about specific herbs and their uses. Moreover, by including individuals with differential knowledge we can distinguish levels of interaction through which information is exchanged and herbs are procured. In turn, the interactions at various levels contribute to the maintenance of similarity of medicinal practices over the area. It is my intention to delineate these hierarchies and levels of interaction through a discussion of disease concepts and herbs, their distribution, and uses.

KNOWLEDGE HIERARCHY OF MEDICINAL BELIEFS AND PRACTICES

Medicinal beliefs are intimately associated with ideas about the nature of the world. Disease concepts of Hispanic America range from those based on witchcraft, evil eye, or bad air to those claiming emotional origin, or organ displacement. Perhaps the most important ideas for our purposes are the belief in the balance of Nature and the fatalistic belief that "God's will" always prevails. The Hispano world consists of elements in balance: rich and poor, sacred and profane, light and dark, hot and cold. In order to remain in balance with one's surroundings one must do things in moderation so as not to disturb the balance. Illness may result when one's relationship with his external environment is altered abruptly, as when experiencing a shock or fright, as well as when one's body's internal balance between hot and cold is disturbed. The latter is very important for a study of medicinal plants as it underlies the system of classifying remedies as hot, cold, or in between -- this is an intrinsic quality of a food or medicine and has little to do with actual temperature. Ailments are also classified as hot or cold and a return to good health is sought through applying the appropriate type of remedy to achieve balance. Simplistically stated, for example, a hot ailment is treated with a cold remedy. Finally, belief in "God's will" as the ultimate cause of illness does not preclude efforts to help one feel better, but it does serve to divert harsh judgement if a cure apparently fails.

Individuals have differential knowlege of ailments and cures as well as disease concepts. From a survey of the literature, and particularly from the author's fieldwork, it became apparent that most adults over the age of 40, and some younger persons, share an acquaintance with the hot-cold classificatory system; that is, they can label some ailments and remedies as hot or cold and know that a hot ailment is treated with a cold remedy. It should be added that how a particular item is classed is highly idiosyncratic but knowing how the classification works facilitates interactions with other persons including curing specialists. Many adults are familiar with common disease concepts -- the specific definitions of which may vary from one locale to another -- such as evil eye (mal de ojo). This is usually a non-malicious, inherent condition of the afflicter which is responsible for certain symptoms, especially in children. Adults outside the immediate family or living unit are careful not to stare at a child, lest they arouse suspicions should the child become ill. Susto or espanto (fright) is a disease concept which many know about -- a frightening episode may cause an anxious emotional state which in turn produces symptoms such as breathing difficulties or stomach gas. Bad air (mal aire or aigre) is widely defined as too much heat or cold invading the body, sometimes from exposure to a dusty whirlwind or other unusual movement of air. This produces various symptoms such as facial twisting, tics, paralysis, dizziness, and headaches. Parents know that babies often suffer from fallen fontanel (caida de mollera), a state in which the fontanel is depressed from vigorous handling or exposure to cold air and the infant is quite ill. Children, and sometimes adults, are known to become afflicted with empacho, a condition in which blockage occurs, causing swelling, bloating and general gastrointestinal distress. This is often attributed to eating too much of certain foods, especially cold foods when one is hot from hard work or play. While laymen may not know specifics of diagnosis or treatment, they are familiar with these diseases and the underlying assumptions like the hot-cold continuum. When a disease such as the above mentioned is suspected they will usually seek the aid of a curing specialist, while minor ailments will be treated at home.

At least a small number of herbal cures, magical charms, and ways to enlist the aid of saints are known to many, if not all, adults. Just as many Anglo-Americans have aspirin, cold tablets, stomach remedies, cough drops, rubbing alcohol, and Bandaids in their medicine cabinets, many Hispanos keep rose petals (Rosa de Castilla -- Rosa spp.) for sore throats, manzanila (Matricaria spp. or Athemis sp.) for stomach upsets and colds, oshá (Ligusticum Porteri) for cuts, inmortal (Asclepias capricornu) for various ailments, and alhucema (Lavandula sp.) for infants' stomachaches. Since the hot-cold classification does not really separate food from medicine, the kitchen is a natural extension of the medicine cabinet. The following items are useful for medicinal purposes: papas (potato slices) and nuez (nutmeg) for headache, canela (cinnámon) for headache and stomachache, albaca (sweet basil) for stomachache, and clavos (cloves) for toothache. Many persons know about and may carry charms such as oshá to keep snakes away, inmortal for luck in love, cachana (Liatris punctata) to protect against witches, and various religious medals.

Beyond the almost universal medical kit described above, virtually every extended family has an older member, generally a woman in most of the area considered here, who knows considerably more about specific symptoms and cures, and her advice is sought when a relative is ill. This individual usually knows several different remedies to try for a particular complaint and where to obtain these if they are not already collected and prepared for use. In the event of a more serious or a chronic ailment, help outside the family may be sought. Neighbors who have more or different remedies to offer are called upon and eventually a person recognized more widely as a specialist may be consulted.

Specialists, known as médicas in northen New Mexico and curanderas in much of the remaining area under study, know considerably more about curing than the average villager as a result of one or more of the following: wider contacts, training by relatives who are (or were) specialists, or possession and use of published pharmacopoeias. Different types of specialists include in New Mexico, for example, a male (médico) specialist who often treats by massage and may be known as a solvador, or a woman specialist (médica) who may also be an accomplished midwife (paterna), although a woman may learn midwifery without becoming a specialist in other aspects of medicine. A specialist often is obvious as such because she or he is paid for goods, e.g., herbs, and services rendered. Some specialists in curing may also be considered witches (brujas) and most curers treat witchcraft-induced ailments; however, brujas often are not curers at all. Curing specialists in all areas utilize religious beliefs and practices to some extent but in certain areas they are involved in spiritualist practices (cf. Kelly 1965, Madsen 1965) and are affiliated with religious sects other than the folk Catholicism of the majority. While many individuals need not leave their home village or a neighboring village, some will travel considerable distances to seek curers of great reputation in another village or in an urban center.

Curing specialists have greater knowledge of and are generally more articulate about disease theory and more adept at diagnosing ailments resulting from fright or evil eye, for example, than other people. While classification of ailments and herbal remedies into hot, cold,or in between categories may be idiosyncratic to the extent that whether an item is hot or cold may vary from one specialist to another, the specialist, in comparison with others, can place items quickly and confidently into categories and use the system extensively in diagnosis and treatment. Specialists utilize more herbs than the average householder and their recipes for medicines are at times quite complicated and may require a number of ingredients, including herbs and other items, plus precise procedures to follow in regard to treatment. Many descriptions of these recipes and treatments are to be found in the literature (Clark 1964, Madsen 1965, Kelly 1965) and are not our concern here. What is important for this study and should be emphasized is that the médicas represent the high point of the knowledge and usage hierarchy and are important nodes in a communication network that disseminates herbal knowledge.

In conclusion it is instructive to note that in proceeding up the hierarchy of knowledge and usage, one finds first an individual with an ailment and perhaps a single plant remedy; his relative or neighbor may suggest one or two alternative plants to try; a specialist will often prescribe an exotic mixture of herbs.

LEVELS OF INTERACTION

Within this situation, where there exists a vast amount of medicinal herb information known collectively by individuals, as well as differential knowledge among individuals, we can distinguish several levels of interaction through which knowledge is exchanged and herbs procured. To better understand the spread of curing information and especially the spatial distribution of herbs it is useful to consider levels of personal interaction. These were alluded to in the previous section where mention was made of the strategy employed when an individual suffered from an ailment.

Individual villagers interact with relatives and other nonspecialists as well as with médicas within their own village, in neighboring villages, and in urban centers. They also interact with priests who are frequently of nonlocal origin and may reside in and serve one village or may travel to several. Peddlers have long been present, especially in the southwestern United States, and often have provided relatively isolated villages with goods, including plants, and information originating from some distance away. In Mexico, markets offer a place for people to meet to exchange herbal curing information and to purchase herbs and other items for treatment. Finally, in the absence of markets, stores such as general stores and drugstores have become an important locus of herbs and curing information in the Southwest.*

A more detailed look at herb sources, procurement, and distribution can be made by examining the potential contacts of an individual Hispano New Mexican. An adult, as mentioned previously, will have some knowledge of remedies for common ailments. Some of these may require such items as tax stamps from cigarette packs (to treat headache), but those requiring plants or plant products may be acquired in various ways. In and around the village he may collect wild herbs such as rosa de Castilla (Rosa spp., rose petals, for sore throat), caña agria (Rumex hymenosepalus, roots, for teeth and gums), chimaja

* In Mexico, too, various stores are outlets for herbs, but I have not personally studied these.

(Cymopterus spp., roots for food, leaves for stomachache as well as seasoning), malvas (Malvas spp., stems and leaves for childbirth and infants), poléo (Hedeoma nanum, stems and leaves for fever), yerba buena (Mentha spicata, stems and leaves for stomachache). Persons with gardens often plant from seed or transplant various herbs for home use including marrubio (Marrubium vulgare), yerba buena, poléo, albaca, oregano (Monarda menthaefolia), altamisa (Artemisia franserioides or Tanacetum vulgare), azafrán (Carthamus tinctorius), cilantro (Coriandrum sativum), and occasionally oshá. Picnics in the mountains are a very popular recreation and provide convenient access to wild herbs native to higher elevations, usually some distance from house and garden, as well as herbs that grow in greater abundance in these locales. Sabina macho (Juniperus communis, needles and berries for urinary disorders), and the aforementioned oshá, altamisa, and oregano are often gathered on these occasions.

Other herbs are more often purchased from peddlers, travelers, or from stores in the form of bundles of plant parts or seeds to plant: oshá, inmortal, contrayerba (Kallstroemia californica), cachana, yerba del manso (Anemopis californica), punche (Nicotiana rustica), manzanilla, alhucema, cáscara sagrada (Rhamnus californica), ruda (Ruta graveolen). romero (Rosmarinus officinalis), te de sena (Cassia sp.). Of these, only the first five are locally available wild, and in fact, stores import others from considerable distances. In the past, peddlers carried these latter items up the Rio Grande from Mexico.

Friends or relatives who travel can often be important sources for herbs -- there is frequent contact between the people of northern New Mexico and those of Mexico. One example of this is a woman, not a médica, native of Nueva Leon who lives in northern New Mexico. When she visits her family in Mexico, she takes orders for herbs from friends in northern New Mexico, fills them through an herb dealer, and brings them back to her friends. The herbs are packaged in brown paper bags with notations as to the ailment which the contents of each should cure. A few individuals order specific herbs, such as azahar (Citris sp.), but most only ask her to get something that is good for a particular ailment and then reorder if they are satisfied. It is my impression that many people in northern New Mexico know someone, perhaps even an anthropologist, who travels to Mexico on occasion and will purchase herbs for them. This type of interaction is not uncommon.

In Mexico the markets are an important source of herbs and curing information as people meet there regularly to buy and sell food, household items, and medicinal herbs. Herb vendors usually are quite knowledgeable about curing, but generally are not considered curanderos. One vendor may sell many different items, fresh in season or dried. An example is a man who has a stall in the Mercado Cuauatemoc in Juarez, Chihuahua (see Appendix D). On the occasion of a visit in May, 1965, he had available nearly 150 herbs as well as a number of patent medicines. In a 10 minute period he made at least 10 sales. Of the 150 herbs, approximately 30 are commonly used in northern New Mexico. Most of these are known by the same name in both locations but a few are known by the dealer to have more than one name, e.g., yerba del manzo = babiza, oshá = chuchupate. The vendor provided uses for most of the herbs and could prescribe when asked. Vendors in markets generally could be considered low level specialists but probably lack the knowledge of a curandera and seldom offer exotic mixtures or complex procedures. Furthermore, they are not really sanctioned as curers within the community and would not be consulted for diagnoses.

Market situations such as this are not generally found in the United States, although individual entrepeneurs do seize opportunities such as fiestas and art fairs to sell herbs. In the Southwest, stores, especially drug stores, have become very important sources of herbal medicines in small towns as well as in the cities of the area as urbanization has tended to remove many people from rural living and the plant world. Drugstores and general stores obtain herbs from various sources. Many buy stock from local collectors and cultivators and mail order from specialty companies. Stores are herb sources for ordinary individuals as well as specialists and often a clerk, pharmacist, or other employee has considerable knowledge of herbal curing, and can assist a customer with purchases appropriate to his or her ailment. While many stores, such as San Juan Mercantile of San Juan Pueblo, New Mexico (until July 1973 when it was destroyed by fire), and Fairview Pharmacy of Española, have only a few herbs for sale, others carry a large supply. Among these are Ruppe's drugstore in Albuquerque (White 1941, see Appendix C), which carried at least 23 herbs in 1941, Pueblo Drug and Valley Drugs in Española, New Mexico, which carry 60-80 different herbs, and a few, such as Tienda de la Salud in Santa Fe, which specialize in herbs to the extent that all other merchandise is secondary to the herbal business. Perhaps the best known of these stores was Roybal's Store, 1917-1968 (see Appendix E). In addition to drugstores, health food stores, flourishing especially since the late 1960s, carry herbs. Thus an individual need not plant or collect his own herbs for medicine as the most common and popular ones are readily available for purchase. These stores serve many individuals over a wide area bounded roughly by Taos on the north, Las Vegas on the east, Jemez Springs on the west, and Albuquerque on the south. They are a very important locus of distribution for herbs and curing knowledge.

CONCLUDING COMMENTS

Interaction of individuals in many different situations accounts for the exchange of information and herbs over a wide area and up and down the hierarchy. A brief discussion about the efficacy of the remedies, the need for different strategies of herb procurement, and the acceptance of new curing information is appropriate. One could list many different remedies for any one common ailment such as stomachache. This is the case for a number of reasons, and if one item is not available, because it is out of season, or climatic conditions are inappropriate, another can be used. If one item does not cure, an alternative can be tried; if one cure helps somewhat, two or three might be even better. Or, if a remedy fails to cure, the diagnosis may be in error. Also, conveniently, the religious belief that "God's will" prevails means that if an ailment fails to be cured by a particular remedy, it does not prove the inefficacy of the herb but only the stubbornness of the ailment, i.e., God wills that one be sick. Meanwhile, it is useful to try anything that might help one to feel better. A further result of this belief is that curing specialists are not generally boycotted for an occasional failure to effect a cure. (It should also be noted that renowned curers select patients with care and often refuse to treat hopeless cases.) Moreover, while few, if any, herbs do harm when properly used (except in occasional cases where their use delays the acquisition of other essential medical aid), there is no doubt that many herbal remedies contain essential nutrients including minerals and vitamins, which very likely assist in the acquisition of good health. Other plants may have value as drugs in the Western medical sense but few have been investigated to determine their pharmacological properties. While some ailments may alleviate without treatment, herbal remedies aid the healing process through physiological and psychological means.

The personal testimony of a friend is sufficient reason to accept a new remedy. Shared disease concepts offer an avenue of acceptance, i.e., if two persons understand evil eye sickness, then one can often convince the other to use a new remedy. Shared classifications such as hot-cold serve similarly as when an individual recognizes he is suffering a stomachache from eating cold foods, another person may convince him to try an unfamiliar herb if the former classifies it as hot and therefore potentially efficacious for a cold ailment. Thus shared beliefs allow new remedies to be accepted and the many loci of interaction keep the information moving, potentially increasing and expanding herbal knowledge and use among individuals at any level of the hierarchy.

In conclusion, it may seem incongruous that in this day of modern medicine folk cures are still popular. In fact, the presence of medical facilities in urban areas does not guarantee use and the inability of professional medical practitioners to attract and deal effectively with the Hispano population in the United States helps perpetuate folk medicine. Western medicine lacks cures for folk diseases, and for common ailments such as colds as well as serious, often fatal diseases, such as cancer and heart disease. There is not only still a place for herbal remedies, but they should not be treated with indifference or condecension by the medical profession. Rather, they should be better understood and accepted as supplementary, complementary, or even substitute treatments. Interestingly, there is also an interest among some educated individuals (several middle-aged women of my acquaintance) in collecting and preserving herbal curing information from relatives both as a hobby and for potential pecuniary reward via possible sale of published material or from the discovery of new miracle drugs extracted from local plants. Finally, the past few years have witnessed a growing trend toward the use of "natural" foods and medicines among non-Spanish individuals, especially Anglos, some of whom live in communes. While this may be of little or no consequence on the Mexican side of the border, this interest and use may favor the continued use of medicinal herbs among all ethnic groups in the southwestern United States for an indefinite period.

APPENDIX A

The Volney H. Jones Collection
Juarez, Chihuahua, 1932

While in the Southwest United States on a plant collecting trip for the Ethnobotanical Laboratory of the University of Michigan, Volney H. Jones purchased economic plants at the market in Juarez. Items were obtained for the comparative collections at the University of Michigan. Jones purchased specimens from five or six dealers and obtained data about usage through an interpreter. Upon his return to Ann Arbor, he catalogued them and identified them botanically when possible. This information appears on the following pages. Appendix D also pertains to Juarez and the comparison is interesting.

Spanish Name	Botanical Name	Catalog Number	Specimen	Use
1. Amole	unidentified	14121	no specimen	Washing hair or clothes: dissolve in hot water
2. Anise	Pimpinella (anisum?)	14118	seeds	Wine making; on bread
3. Bavisa (see Yerba Mansa)				
4. Cañahuala	Notholaena sinuata var. integerrima Hook.	14115	bundle of plants	Stomach medicine: an infusion is made
5. Cañaigre	Rumex hymenosepalus Torr.	14104	dried roots	Stomach medicine and blood tonic
6. Comino	Cuminum cyminium	14119	fruit	Food: used in sausage
7. Cuasia	?Quassia amara L.	14120	small pieces of wood	Stomach upset from anger: soak in water and drink liquid
8. Frijilito	Erthyrina flabelliformis	14641	beans	
9. Guachichile or Huichichili or Wachichile	Loesilia coccines Brand.	14111	bundle of stems and leaves	Fever and colds: plant used to make tea which is drunk and bathed in

10. Lanten	*Plantago major* L.	14109	stems, leaves, and fruit	Cuts: used as a poultice, wash wounds and then apply
11. Manzanilla	*Matricaria* sp.	14103	bundle of whole plants	Stomach tonic: infusion is made
12. Matariqui	unidentified	14116	roots	Kidney disorders: roots are boiled and the liquid used
13. Nogal	*Juglans* sp.	14117	herbarium specimen	Blood tonic: infusion of the boiled leaves
14. Poléo	*Cunila longiflora*	14112	bundle of herb	Beverage: a drink for babies is made from it
15. Popotillo	*Ephedra antisyphilitica* Meyer	14108	bundle of stems	Stomach medicine: an infusion of the stems is mixed with lemon or orange juice and sugar
16. Romero	unidentified	14113	bundle of herb	
17. Seniso	unidentified	14114	bundle of stems with leaves	Stomach medicine: an infusion is made
18. Tamarind	*Tamarindus indica*	14107	beans of the plant	Beverage: dissolve beans in water and add sugar. Flavoring: e.g., ice cream

Spanish Name	Botanical Name	Catalog Number	Specimen	Use
19. Yerba Mansa	Anemopsis californica (Nutt.) Hook. and Arn.	14110	bundle of plants	Boils: infusion used as a wash
20. Lleva del Sapo	Cirsium undulatum (Nutt.) Spreng.	14102	leaves and flowers	Fever: used for making a drink and for bathing
21. Zacate de limon	Cymbopogon citratus	14105	bundles of grass	Beverage: boil leaves in water
22.	Lippia nodiflora	14106	bundle of stems with leaves	

APPENDIX B

The Lundell and Whiting Collection, 1934

In 1934 the University of Michigan Herbarium conducted an expedition to Mexico. Cyrus Longworth Lundell, then Curator of Phanerogams, and Alfred Whiting, then a graduate student in botany, collected economic plants at Charcas, San Luís Potosí, and Monterrey, Nueva Leon. Food and medicinal plants were obtained in local markets; assistants then helped to find herbarium specimens of the same plants in the field. These specimens are available in the Ethnobotanical Laboratory at The University of Michigan Museum of Anthropology. Lundell and Whiting identified the plants and collected some data on usage. Their notes were used to compile the following charts which list the plants by Spanish name and include the Ethnobotanical Laboratory catalog number, type of specimen, source, and use. In most instances a question mark reflects the notation Whiting and Lundell used on their data sheets. I added a very few question marks in cases where the original source was unclear or illegible. These charts include the complete collection. Many of the items included here are entered in the Spanish-name Glossary (Appendix F). Plants were not included if both usage and Latin name were lacking.

Spanish Name	Botanical Name	Catalog Number	Specimen	Location or Source	Use
1. Agrito	Oxalis albicans H.B.K. (AFW?)	W663	no specimen	Charcas, enclosed hillside	
	Oxalis sp. (AFW?)	W676	no specimen	Charcas, damp ground	
	Pellaea cordata (Cav.) J. Sm. (Maxon)	W752	no specimen	Charcas, mountain side	
	Oxalis leonis	W597	no specimen	Charcas, enclosed hillside	
2. Alamo	unidentified	W943 14913	no specimen	Charcas?	
3. Albacar	Scutellaria	L5656 15108	bundle of whole plants	Monterrey	
4. Alejandria	Cowania plicata D. Don.	L5248 14986	bundles of stems with leaves and flowers	Charcas	
5. Alfalfa	Medicago sativa L. (AFW?)	W569	no specimen	Charcas, enclosed hillside	For (the) heads

6.	Alfilerillo	*Erodium cicutarium* (L.) L'Hér. (C.V. Morton)	W900 14889	mounted pressed whole plant	Charcas, enclosed hillside	Sore throat
		Erodium cicutarium (L.) L'Hér.	W674 14866	pressed whole plant	Charcas, low land once inhabited	Used to make gargle for sore throat
7.	Alfilerillo	*Acalypha hederaceae* Torr. *Erodium cicutarium* (L.) L'Hér.	L5255 14993	mass of roots, stems, leaves	Charcas	Gargle when the throat is closed. Boiled and liquid used
8.	Almorrana	unidentified	L5618 15069	bundle of stems with leaves, flowers and pressed whole plant	Monterrey	Medicinal herb
9.	Alta Misa	*Zaluzania triloba* (Ort.) Pers. (AFW?)	W725 14870 L5357	pressed whole plant without root	Charcas plain	
		Zaluzania triloba (Ort.) Pers. (AFW?)	W767 L5357		West of San Diego	

Spanish Name	Botanical Name	Catalog Number	Specimen	Location or Source	Use
	Zaluzania triloba (Ort.) Pers. (AFW?)	W867 14881 L5357		Charcas plain	
10. Altimisa	Parthenium lyratum Gray (AFW?)	W671 L5206		Charcas land once inhabited	
	unidentified	L5717 15170	bundle of stems with leaves, flowers		
11. Altamisa del Campo	Franseria confertifolia Parthenium lyratum	L5695b 15147	bundles of stems with leaves, flowers		
12. Altamisa de Castilla		L5028 14948	all but root	Saltillo	Stomachache
13. Alurema (Alucema?)	Lavandula sp.	L5647 15098	flowers	Monterrey	
14. Amapola	Galpinsia hortwegi (Benth.) Britton (AFW?) also identified as Oenothera Greggii var. Pringelei Munz. (C.V. Morton)	W898 14887 also L5125	pressed whole plant without root	Charcas, enclosed hillside	Boil in water good for cough

	unidentified	W566		Charcas, enclosed hillside	Boil in water, good for cough
	Galpinsia hartwegi (Benth.) Britton	L5125 (W898)	all but root	Charcas	Boil in water, good for cough
15. Amargo	unidentified	W5247 14985	pieces of roots	Charcas	Medicinal plant
16. Amarrio	*Prunus armeniaca* (L) (CLL)	W947 14917		Orchard near Charcas	Small, round, yellow edible fruit
17. Angrelitas	*Houstonia acerosa* Gray (C.V. Morton)	W911 14895	mounted pressed whole plant	Charcas, enclosed hillside	Good for restrained urine
18. Anis Chico	*Pimpinella anisum*	L5639 15090	seeds	Monterrey	
19. Apio	unidentified	L5567 15056	stems, leaves also, pressed whole plant	Charcas	For bathing: boil in water and bathe with water; good for inflammation, ?neuralgia
		L5610 15061	bundle of stems with leaves, pressed plant	Monterrey	Boiled. Food and medicinal herb

Spanish Name	Botanical Name	Catalog Number	Specimen	Location or Source	Use
20. Arnica	<u>Aplopappus</u> <u>spinulosus</u> var. <u>turbinellus</u> (Rydb) Blake	L5675 15127	several whole plants		
	<u>Grindelia</u> <u>oxylepis</u> Greene	L5269a 15007	bundles of whole plant		
	<u>Gaillardia</u> <u>nervosa</u> Rydb. (S.F. Blake)	W912 14896		Charcas, enclosed hillside	Flowers in alcohol for wound
	<u>Gaillardia</u> <u>nervosa</u> Rydb. (AFW?)	W679		Charcas, enclosed hillside	For wounds
	<u>Gaillardia</u> <u>Mervosa</u> Rydb. (AFW?) (sic)	W790		Plateau west San Diego	For curing wounds; the flowers are placed in alcohol
21. Artizuilla or Artiguilla	<u>Bouteloua</u> <u>gracilis</u> (H.B.K.) Lag. (A.S. Hitchcock)	W672		Charcas, lowland	
22. Azahar de Naranjo	<u>Citris</u> (<u>C</u>. <u>sinensis</u>?)	L5632 15083	flower petals	Monterrey	Flowers of a citris

23. Barba de Chivo	Clematis Drumondii T. and G. (AFW?)	W661		Charcas, enclosed hillside	Leaves used for excited animals
	Clematis Drummondii (C.V. Morton)	W906 14894	pressed plant with stem, leaves, flower	Charcas, enclosed hillside	For skin eruptions a small leaf is held between the fingers and rubbed on the skin. Also for curing animals, small leaf and beat with water, and apply
24. Barba de Coco	Cocos nucifera L.	L5568 15057	fruit husk	Charcas	Medicinal
25. Benna Dia	Porophyllum filiforme Rydb. (S.F. Blake)	W921 14905	pressed plant with stems, leaves, flowers	Charcas, rocky slope	Boil in water as substitute for castor oil. Laxative
26. Betonia	unidentified	L5716 15169	bundle of stems with leaves, flowers	Monterrey	Medicinal herb

Spanish Name	Botanical Name	Catalog Number	Specimen	Location or Source	Use
27. Bogambilia	Bougainvillea spectabilis	L5614 15065	leaves	Monterrey	For cough, boiled with other herbs
28. Bolitas Quasima	Guazuma ulmifolia	L5702 15154	seedpods	Monterrey	Medicinal for gonorrhea
29. Borraja	Borago officinale	L5412 15027	bundles of stems with leaves, flowers	Charcas	
	Borago officinale	L5682 15134	bundles of stems with leaves, flowers	Monterrey	Fever medicine
	Sonchus oleraceus L. (AFW?)	W574 L5080		Charcas, enclosed hillside	
30. Brazíl	5 names listed: Caesalpinia crista Condalia obovata Haematoxylum brasiletto H. campechianum H. Boreale	L5652b 15104	vial of small chips of wood		

31. Bura Dulce	*Eysenhardtia polystachya* (Orteg.) Sarg. (CLL)	W550 L5128		Charcas shrub	
32. Cabesona	unidentified	L5704 15156	bundles of whole plants		
33. Cachan	unidentified	L5700 15152	several roots		
34. Calabasa	*Cucurbita* sp. (C.V. Morton)	W1005 14922		Charcas market	Flowers for soup
	C. muschata (M.R. Gilmore)	W1006 14923		Charcas market	Squash fruit to eat
35. Calampacate	*Gnaphalium semiamplexicaule* LC. (CLL)	W920 14904		San Diego	Leaf placed over a wound
36. Canaguala	fern	L5687 15139	bundle of stems with leaves and pressed plant	Monterrey	Medicinal herb
37. Candeliya or Candelilla	unidentified	L5216 14954	bundles of stems and pressed plant	Charcas	For bladder trouble

Spanish Name	Botanical Name	Catalog Number	Specimen	Location or Source	Use
38. Capitanejo	unidentified	L5416 15031	bundles of stems with leaves and pressed plant	Charcas	For washing wounds and boils of animals
39. Carcoma	*Milla biflora* Cav. (C.V. Morton)	W492		Charcas, protected hillside	Bulb eaten
40. Cardo Santo	*Argemone platyceras* Link and Otto (AFW)	W571		Charcas, enclosed hillside	
41. Cebada	*Hordeum vulgare* L.	W605		Charcas, near corn field	
42. Cebollita del Campo	*Allium scaposum* Benth.	W764		Charcas, near corn field	
43. Cedro	*Cupressus benthamii* Encl1. (CLL)	W587 L5166		Charcas	Cultivated
44. Cedron	*Lippia triphylla* (L'Hér.) Kuntze (CLL)	W585 14854 L5167	pressed plant with stem, leaves, flowers	Charcas	For colic in women, boil in water

45. Cedron de Castilla	*Lippia triphylla* (L'Hér.) Kuntze	L5025 14945	bundle of stems with leaves	Saltillo	Boiled and taken as a drink in treating colic
	Lippia triphylla (L'Hér.) Kuntze	L5418 15033	bundles of stems with leaves and pressed plant	Charcas	For colic, boiled and taken for colic mixed with Muicle
	Lippia triphylla (L'Hér.) Kuntze	L5649 15100	bundle of stems with leaves and pressed plant	Monterrey	For colic
46. Charrsas-quilla	unidentified	L5705 15158	bundle of thorny stems with leaves and flowers	Monterrey	
47. Chia	unidentified	W940 14910		Charcas, broken ground	
48. Chili Perrana, Chili, Chili Cascabel	*Capsicum frutescens* L. Cayenne Group (AFW)	W1008 14925		Charcas market	

Spanish Name	Botanical Name	Catalog Number	Specimen	Location or Source	Use
49. Chili Verde	*Capsicum frutescens* L. Perfection Group (AFW)	W1007 14924		Charcas market	Soup and flavoring
50. Chilito Pajarito	unidentified	W914 14898	pressed root, stem and seeds	Charcas, enclosed hillside	
51. Cilantro	*Coriandrum sativum* (AFW)	W1004 14921		Charcas market	For flavoring soup
52. Cimonillo	unidentified	W5249 14987 L5349b	bundles of whole plants few roots and pressed plant	Charcas	To give appetite
53. Cinco Yagay	*Tagetes* sp.	L5242 14980	dry stems with an occasional root	Charcas	
54. Contra Yerba	*Psoralea pentophylla* L. (C.V. Morton)	W870 14884	pressed whole plant without root	Plateau near San Diego	Root peeled and eaten for stomach trouble

55. Contrayerba	list of 10 names likely -- Psoralea pentaphylla (W870)	L5224 14962	small roots strung together		
56. Copal Goma	unidentified	L5643b 15094	small rocks in vial		
57. Corteza de Alamo Blanco	Populus sp.	L5415 15030	pieces of bark	Charcas	
58. Corteza de Mesquite	unidentified	L5654 15106	strips of bark	Monterrey	
59. Costomate	Physalis ?costomall pubescen.	W1088 14937	pieces of roots	Charcas	
	Physalis ?pubescens	L5250 14988	bundles of stems	Charcas	
60. Crespa	unidentified	L5691 15143	stems with leaves and flowers	Monterrey	Medicinal
61. Cuacia	unidentified	W1089 14938 see 5251	chips of wood		
62. Culantrillo	Adiantum capillus veneris L.	L5651 15102	bundles of stems with leaves	Monterrey	Boiled medicinal herb

Spanish Name	Botanical Name	Catalog Number	Specimen	Location or Source	Use
	Adiantum capillus veneris L.	L5422 15037	bundles of stems with leaves	Charcas	For retarded period in women. Boiled in water and taken
63. Drago	Pterocarpus acapulceusis Rose	L5664 15116	roots	Monterrey	
64. Durazno	unidentified	W946 14916		Orchard near Charcas	Small, round, green fruit eaten
65. Egara	Picus carica (L) (CLL)	W942 14912		Charcas	Eat fruit
66. Ensino	Quercus sp. ?	L5665 15117	pieces of bark	Monterrey	For loose teeth
67. Escobilla	Buddleia scordiodes H.B.K. (CLL)	W649 L5138		Charcas, enclosed hillside	Good for indigestion or empacho, boiled in water
68. Escobillo	Buddleia scordiodes H.B.K. (CLL)	W939 L5138 14909		Charcas, enclosed hillside	Stomach trouble. Boiled in water

69. Escobillo salvilla	*Buddleia scordiodes* H.B.K.	L5238 14976	bundles of stems with leaves and flowers	Charcas	Constipation and bad stomach
70. Espanto Vaquero	*Ipomoea* sp.	L5218 14956	several chunks of root	Charcas	Kidney and urinary troubles. Pains in the shoulder
	Ipomoea sp.	L5434b 15049	a large root	Charcas	For kidneys and lungs
	Ipomoea sp.	L5434 15049	bundles of stems with leaves and flowers	Charcas	For kidneys and lungs
	Ipomea sp. (AFW)	W549 14853	flower	Charcas, inhabited area	
71. Estafiate see also Istafiate	unidentified	W785		West San Diego shrub	Good for susto and fright
72. Estoraque	unidentified	L5643c 15094	vial of rocks		
73. Estrella del norte	*Asphodelus fistulosus* L. (C.V. Morton)	W567		Charcas, enclosed hillside	

Spanish Name	Botanical Name	Catalog Number	Specimen	Location or Source	Use
74. Eucalita	Eucaluptus sp.	L5619 15070	leaves	Monterrey	With other herbs for cough
75. Fistola	unidentified	L5626 15077	seed pod		
76. Flor de Acocotiyo or Acocotillo	?Arracacia atro-purpureus Anethum foeniculum Foeniculum: Conium	L5417 15032 L5638 15089	seeds bigger seeds		
77. Flor Altea	Hibiscus syriacus	L5621 15072	flowers	Monterrey	Medicinal herb (cough)
78. Flor de Bougainbilla	Bougainvillea spectabilis	L5430 15045	flowers and leaves	Charcas	For cough: boiled and drunk
79. Flor de Cananita	unidentified	L5413 15029	flowers in packets		
80. Flor de Cardo Santo	Cirsium undulatum Gray	L5431a L5431b 15046	flowers	Charcas	
	Centaurea americana Nutt.	L5636 15087	flowers	Monterrey	

81. Flor de Castilla	_Rosa_ sp. (_R_. _Centifolia_?)	L5254 14992	flowers	Charcas	Flowers of cultivated rose (?). Boiled and liquid used for enema
82. Flor de un Dia	_Sanvitalia ocymoides_ D.C.	L5425 15040	bundles of whole plants	Charcas	
83. Flor de Lita	_Melia azedarach_? _Pithosporum tobira_ _Syringa vulgaris_ L.	L5627 15078	leaves, flowers	Monterrey	
84. Flor de Manzanilla	unidentified	L5253 14991	flowers		
85. Flor de Mimbre	5 names listed: _Acacia perlandieri_ _Cephalanthus salifolium_ _Chilopsis linearis_ _Forestiera_ (?) _tomentosa_ _Capparis flexnosa_	L5225 see L5661 14963	flowers		
86. Flor de Nacahiula	_Cordia boisieri_ (sp?)	L5646 15097	flowers and a few leaves	Monterrey	
87. Flor de Palma, or Flor de Palma Chino	_Yucca_ sp.	L5276 15014	flowers	Charcas	For strong cough

Spanish Name	Botanical Name	Catalog Number	Specimen	Location or Source	Use
88. Flor de Peña	Selaginella	L5409 15024	whole plant	Charcas	
89. Flor de San Juan	Bouvardia longiflora	L5421 15036	flowers on stems with some leaves		
	Macrosiphonia apocinas hypoleaca (?)	L5667 15119	flowers		
90. Flor sauco	Sambucus mexicana Presl	L5629 15080	flowers	Monterrey	For cough, used with other herbs
91. Flor de Saugua	Sambucus mexicana Presl	L5024 14944	bundles of stems with leaves, flowers	Saltillo	To relieve cough
92. Garavatillo	Mimosa biuncifera Benth. (CLL)	W648 L5141		Charcas, enclosed hillside	
93. Gobernadora	Larrea tridentata (D C.) Coville (CLL)	W726 L5298 14871	pressed, stem (branch) with leaves flowers	Charcas, plain shrub	For the stomach: boil and drink

94. Gobernadora	*Larrea tridentata* (DC) Coville	L5661a 15113	bundles of stems with leaves and flowers	Monterrey	
	Larrea tridentata (DC) Coville	L5230 14968	bundles of stems with leaves and flowers	Charcas	Market herb. Medicinal
95. Golondrina	*Dichondra argentea* H.B.K.	W639 14859	pressed stems with leaves and flowers	Charcas, enclosed hillside	For all kinds of pains in the stomach: boil in water
	Euphorbia sp.	L5228 14966	bundles of stems with leaves and flowers	Charcas	Medicinal herb
	Euphorbia	L5622 15073	bundles of stems with leaves and flowers	Monterrey	Medicinal herb
96. Gordolobo	*Gnaphalium semi-amplexicaule*	L5256 14994	bundles of stems with leaves and flowers	Charcas	Gargles, cough

Spanish Name	Botanical Name	Catalog Number	Specimen	Location or Source	Use
	Gnaphalium sp.	L5648 15099	bundles of stems with leaves and flowers	Monterrey	Medicinal herb
97. Gordo Lobo	identification not practical, possible Eupa-torium or Brickellia	W918 14902	mounted root stem, leaves, package of (seeds?)	San Diego	No use known to informant
98. Grama	Family: Grami-neae	L5217 14955	bundles of whole plants and pressed plant	Charcas	Urinary system
99. Grangene	Ephedra aspera Engelm. (AFW?)	W607		Charcas, transect A	
100. Granjano	unidentified	W713		Charcas, plain shrub	
101. Guaccimas	Guazuma ulmifolia	L5223 14961	seedpods	Charcas	For urinary troubles. Boiled with other herbs

102. Guachichile	*Loesilia coccinea* Brand	L5220 14958	bundles of stems with leaves and flowers	Charcas	
	Loesilia coccinea Brand	L5655 15107	bundles of stems with leaves and flowers	Monterrey	
103. Guachi-chiligo	*Loeselia coerulea* Don	L5426 15041	bundles of whole plants	Charcas	
104. Guayacan	*Guaiacum Coulteri* *Guaiacum Zigafilas* *Guaiacum guatemalas* Palermi etc.	L5708 15161	large pieces of woody stem some bark peeled off		
105. Gueso de Mamell	*Pithecoctenium echinatum* Schl.	15052	nuts	Charcas	Good for curling hair: grind and beat with vigor and rub in the hair
106. Hinojo	unidentified	L5261 L5261b 14999	bundles of stems with leaves and pressed plant	Charcas	To cause sweat in bathing. Used with other herbs.

Spanish Name	Botanical Name	Catalog Number	Specimen	Location and Source	Use
		15099	bundle of stems, leaves		To cause sweat in bathing. Used with other herbs
		L5684 15138	stems and leaves	Monterrey	Medicinal
107. Hojas de Nogal	_Juglans_ sp.	L5408 15023	bundles of stems with leaves and pressed plant	Charcas	To increase or give strengh to the blood
108. Hojas de Sen	List of 3 names: _Caesalpinia exo-stemma_ DC. _Cassia covesii_ Gray _Flourensia cernua_ DC.	L5641 15092	leaves		
109. Hojase	_Flourensia cernua_ DC.	L5244 14982	bundles of stems with leaves and flowers	Charcas	
	Flourensia cernua DC.	L5674 15126	bundles of stems with leaves and flowers		

110. Huisache	Acacia farnesiana (L.) Willd. (CLL)	W915 L5190 14899		Charcas, enclosed hillside	The mature fruit contains ink which can be used for writing
111. Incienso	unidentified	L5643d 15094	little rocks in vial		
112. Indio	Aristolochia anguisida Aristolochia foelida (sp??)	W1087 14936	pieces of root		
113. Ineldo	Anethum graveolens	L5694 15146	bundle of stems with leaves and seeds	Monterrey	
114. Injerto de Mésquite or Grijente de Mesquite	unidentified	L5681 15133	stems and leaves		
115. Ipasote de Comer	unidentified	L5670b 15122	bundle of whole plants without roots and pressed plant	Monterrey	Medicinal herb

Spanish Name	Botanical Name	Catalog Number	Specimen	Location or Source	Use
116. Ipasote Sarrillo	Chenopodium sp.	L5259 14997	bundles of stems and flowers	Charcas	For chills after getting wet. Boil and drink.
117. Istafiate	Artemisia mexicana Willd.	L5243 14981	bundles of whole plants	Charcas	Toasted, powdered, and given to babies mixed with breast milk
	Artemisia	L5673 15125	bundles of stems with leaves and flowers		
118. Itamo Rial	Ephedra aspera Engelm.	L5215 14953	bundles of stems	Charcas	Bladder trouble. Boiled with other herbs
119. Jasmin	unidentified	L5713 15166	flowers		
120. Javonsillo or Jaronsillo	Parosela caudata Rydb. (CLL)	W565		Charcas, enclosed hillside	

121. Judica?	unidentified	L5263 15001	bundles of stems with leaves and a few flowers	Charcas	For bath to cause sweat and fried in grease and applied to wounds
122. Lanten	<u>Plantago</u> <u>major</u> L.	L5235 14973	bundles of stems with leaves and flowers (seeds)	Charcas	For constipa- tion
123. Laurel	<u>Litsea</u> <u>pringlei</u> Bartlett	L5428 15043	stems (branches) with leaves	Charcas	Medicinal herb
124. Leihuguilla Mansa	<u>Agave</u> <u>perplexans</u> (Trelease)	W832		Plain below Mt. Aguila	For washing as with soap: the root is used for washing clothes, dishes and one's self
125. Lengua de Vaca	<u>Rumex</u> <u>mexicanus</u> Meisn. (AFW?)	W705 14869	pressed plant with stem, leaves and flowers	Charcas, in water	
126. Limoncillo	<u>Dyssodia</u> <u>penta-chaeta</u> (DC.) Robinson	L5240 14978	bundles of whole plants	Charcas	For constipa- tion

Spanish Name	Botanical Name	Catalog Number	Specimen	Location or Source	Use
		L5668 15120	bundle of stems with leaves, flowers		
127. Mala Mujer	<u>Solanum</u> <u>rostratum</u>	L5569 15058	bundles of stems with leaves, flowers and pressed plant	Charcas	
128. Malva	unidentified	W675		Charcas	Boiled in water, used in washing wounds
		L5270 15008	bundles of whole plants		
129. Manzanilla del Campo	<u>Zinnia</u> <u>pumila</u> Gray	W733		Charcas	
130. Manzanilla Castilla		L5672 15124	bundle of stems with leaves, flowers and pressed plant	Monterrey	Medicinal herb

131. Manzanilla	unidentified	L5252 14990	bundles of stems with leaves, flowers	Charcas market	Boiled and taken
		L5027 14947	bundle of dry stems with the remains of leaves, flowers	Saltillo market	Colic
132. Manzanilla Loco	unidentified	W897 14886	pressed stems with leaves, flowers	Charcas, enclosed hillside	
133. Mariola	unidentified shrub	W862 14877	pressed stems with leaves, flowers	Charcas plain	
	Parthenium incanum H.B.K.	L5245 14983	bundles of stems with leaves, flowers	Charcas	Bitters, for stomach trouble
	Parthenium incanum H.B.K.	L5690 15142	bundles of stems with leaves, flowers	Monterrey	

Spanish Name	Botanical Name	Catalog Number	Specimen	Location or Source	Use
134. Marrubio	Marrubium vulgare L.	L5696b 15148	bundles of stems with leaves and flowers	Monterrey	
	Marrubium vulgare L. (AFW)	W536		Charcas inhabited area	"For frights"
	Marrubium vulgare L.	W902 14891	pressed whole plant	Charcas, enclosed hillside	For rheumatism, for sleep, for fright. For fright place the plant under mattress.
135. Mejorana	unidentified	L5236 14974	bundles of stems with leaves and pressed	Charcas	For constipation and to give appetite
136. Menta	unidentified	L5659 15111	bundles of whole plants without roots		
137. Mesquite	Prosopis chilensis (Mol.) Stuntz (AFW?)	W655 14863 L5144		Charcas, enclosed hillside	

138. Mimbre	unidentified	L5616 15067	flowers, a few leaves		
139. Mirta Raja	unidentified	L5262 15000	bundles of stems with leaves		
140. Mirto del Campo	unidentified	W537 L5056 14852		Charcas, inhabited area	For biliousness boil in water and drink
141. Mirto de Castilla	<u>Salvia</u>	L5612 15063	bundles of stems with leaves and flowers	Monterrey	Medicinal herb, colic
142. Mirto	<u>Salvia chamae-dryoide</u> Cav. (AFW?)	W673 14865	pressed whole plant	Charcas lowland	For "bilis". Boiled in water
143. Misto	unidentified	W949 14919	pressed stem with leaves, flower	Charcas, mountain base	For "bilis".
144. Misto del Campo	unidentified	W696		Charcas mountain bank or arroya	For "bilis".
145. Moctezuma or Montezuma	unidentified	L5234 14972	bundles of stems with leaves, flowers and pressed plant	Charcas	Rheumatism

Spanish Name	Botanical Name	Catalog Number	Specimen	Location or Source	Use
146. Monasillo	Malvaviscus spp.	L5637 15088	flowers with a few leaves	Monterrey	For cough. Used with other herbs
147. Moradillo	Funastrum heterophyllum (Engelm.) Standl.	L5275 15013	bundles of stems with leaves and flowers	Charcas	Boiled and liquid used to bathe children when they are feverish
148. Mostosa Loca	unidentified	W820		Plateau near Mt. Aguila	
149. Muicle	unidentified	L5419 15034	stems, leaves and pressed plant	Charcas	Medicinal herb
		L5662 15114 L5662b	stems with leaves and flowers and pressed plant	Monterrey	Medicinal herb
150. Mula	Eupatorium subintegrum (Greene) Robinson?	L5699 15151	bundles of stems with leaves and flowers	Monterrey	Medicinal herb

151. (de la) Mula	Eupatorium subintegrum (Greene)	L5233 14971	bundles of stems with leaves	Charcas	Treatment of rheumatism
152. Nogal	Juglans sp.	L5707 15160	pieces of bark and pressed leaves	Monterrey	Medicinal bark
	Juglans sp.	L5707 15160 L5707c	leaves on stems (branches) bark and pressed leaves	Monterrey	Medicinal
153. Neldo	Anethum graveolens L.	15146	whole plant		
154. Nues Mosquiada or Moscada	Myristica sp.	L5645 15096	several whole nuts		
155. Oregano or Salvia	list of Hyptis albida Origanum majorum Origanum vulgare Paliomintha longiflora Calamintha potosina	L5634 15085	leaves, stems and seeds		

Spanish Name	Botanical Name	Catalog Number	Specimen	Location or Source	Use
156. Orejeula de Raton	Dichondra argentea Willd.	L5272 15010	bundles of stems with leaves and flowers	Charcas	To give appetite
157. Orejuela Raton	Dichondra argentea Willd.	L5640 15091	bundles of stems with leaves and flowers	Monterrey	
158. Orteguilla	unidentified	L5718 15171	bundle of stems with leaves and flowers and pressed	Monterrey	Market herb
159. Ortiga (?Orteguilla)	unidentified	L5278 15016	bundles of stems with leaves and a few flowers	Charcas	Medicine
160. Otate	Family Gramineae Tribe Bambuseae	L5414 15029	sticks of woody stem	Charcas, imported from Tula, Tamaulipas	For internal tumors
	Family Gramineae Tribe Bambuseae	L5624 15075	pieces of woody stem	Monterrey	For reducing inflamation

161. "Palmar"	unidentified	W707		Charcas, dominant tree in Yucca mesquite bush	"Palmar" association tree= palma used by natives for wood
162. Palo Azul	Eysenhardtia polystachya	L5611 15062	pieces of woody stem	Monterrey	Medicinal wood
163. Palo Santo	unidentified	L5692 15144	bundle of stems with large leaves	Monterrey	Medicine (leaves crushed, smell like sasafras)
164. Palomas de la Punsada	unidentified	L5280 L5018	large open seedpod with many seeds		
165. Parraleña	Dyssodia setifolia (Lag.) Robinson	L5241 14979	bundles of stems with leaves and flowers and pressed plant	Charcas	For constipation
	Dyssodia setifolia (Lag.) Robinson (S.F. Blake)	W904 14892	pressed whole plant	Charcas, enclosed hillside	For cough -- in water

Spanish Name	Botanical Name	Catalog Number	Specimen	Location or Source	Use
	Gyssodia setifolia (sic) (Lag.) Robinson (AFW?)	W609		Charcas plateau open field	Good for stomachache
166. Paschtle	*Tillandsia recurvata* L. (AFW?)	W506		Charcas, on mesquite	
167. (del) Pasmo	unidentified	L5264 15002	bundles of stems with leaves and pressed plant	Charcas	Fried in grease and applied to bowel region for chills and gas pains
168. Pasmo	unidentified	L5685 15137	bundle of stems with leaves and pressed plant	Monterrey	Medicinal herb
169. Pastle de Mesquite	*Tillandsia recurvata* L. (AFW?)	W738		Charcas on mesquite	
170. Pata de Res	*Cassia bauhinioides* Gray	L5424 15039	bundles of stems with leaves, flowers and seed pods	Charcas	Mild laxative for small children

171. Pata de Vaca	unidentified	L5644b 15095	bundle of stems with leaves, flowers and pressed	Monterrey	Medicinal herb
172. Pata de Ves	*Cassia banhinioides* Gray (AFW?)	W787 L5361 L5345 14873	pressed with stem, leaves, pods, flowers	Plateau west of San Diego	For stomach-ache and "bilis". Boil in water and drink
173. Pazote de Comer	*Chenopodium ambrosioides* L. (C. V. Morton)	W917 14901	pressed whole plant without root	San Diego, Charcas	For a pain. Boiled in water
174. Pega Ropa	*Mentezelia hispida* Willd. (C.V. Morton)	W869 L5161 14883	pressed branch with leaves, flowers	Plateau near San Diego	For urine trouble
	Mentezelia hispida Willd (?)	L5227 14965	roots	Charcas	Medicinal herb. Powdered
175. Perejil	unidentified	L5671 L5671b 15123 15009	bundle of stems with leaves and pressed	Monterrey	For the heart

Spanish Name	Botanical Name	Catalog Number	Specimen	Location or Source	Use
176. Perritos de Huerto	unidentified	W552		Charcas, enclosed hillside	
177. Peston	<u>Eupatorium</u> sp. (AFW?)	W938 14908	pressed stems with leaves	Charcas, enclosed hillside	Stomach trouble Powdered in water.
	<u>Eupatorium</u> sp.	L5237 14975	bundles of stems with leaves and flowers	Charcas	For constipa-tion
178. Piania	<u>Perezia</u> <u>runci-nata</u> Lag.	L5226 14964	whole plant leaves, flowers, stems, roots	Charcas	For chest troubles. Boiled and mixed with other herbs.
179. Picaro	<u>Bidens</u> sp. (AFW?)	W645		Charcas, enclosed hillside	
180. Pichi-chagua	<u>Perezia</u> <u>nana</u> Gray	L5219 14957 2 boxes	whole plant in bundle	Charcas	Urinary sys-tem. Rat poison (when boiled)
181. Pico Pajaro	<u>Lycium</u> <u>Schaffneri</u> Gray (AFW?)	W784 L5355		West of San Diego shrub	

182. Pico de Pajaro	Rhus microphylla Engelm. (AFW?)	W700		San Diego small shrub	
183. Pirul	Schinus molle L	L5693 15145	bundle of stems with leaves	Monterrey	Medicinal herb
184. Poléo de Castilla (Poléo)	unidentified	L5676 15128	bundle of stems with leaves and pressed plant	Monterrey	Medicine
		L5562 15051	bundles of stems with leaves flowers and pressed	Charcas	Medicinal
185. Poléo de Menta (Poléo)	unidentified	L5566 15055	bundles of whole plants without roots		
186. Quassia (Quassia Amara)	Picrasma excelsa? Pecrasinn excelsa (sp?)	L5251 14989	chips of wood		
187. Quina (Copal-quin?)	Chinchana succumbra Coutarea latiflora Coutarea pterosperma	L5711 15164	large pieces of bark		

Spanish Name	Botanical Name	Catalog Number	Specimen	Location or Source	Use
188. Rais de China	Smilax cordifolia	L5709 15162	chunks of roots		
189. Rais de Lipana	unidentified	L5635 15086	several roots		
190. Ramon	Parosela canescens (Mart and Gal) Rose	W678 L5328 14867	pressed branch with leaves	Charcas bank of arroya	For regulating the stomach
191. Romerillo	unidentified	W551		Charcas inhabited area	
192. Romero	unidentified	L5023 14961	bundle of branches with leaves and pressed	Saltillo market	Stomachaches
	Rosmarinus officinalis L.?	L5281 15019	a few leaves, some pressed	Charcas	Burned in houses to chase out snakes and obnoxious insects

		L5695c 15147	bundle of stems with leaves flowers and pressed stems and leaves	Monterrey	Medicinal herb
193.	Rosa de Castilla	Rosa sp. (R. centifolia?)	L5630 15081	flowers	Monterrey	Medicinal herb
194.	Rosita	Gutierrezia sarothrae (Pursh) Britt. and Brown (AFW?)	W563		Charcas, enclosed hillside	
195.	Ruda	unidentified	L5277 L5277b L5715 5715b 15015 15168	bundles of stems with leaves, flowers and pressed plant	Monterrey	Headache -- To let the air out of the head
196.	Sacasil	?Anredera scandens Moge ?Boussingaultia baselloides HBK	15082	?fruits		

Spanish Name	Botanical Name	Catalog Number	Specimen	Location or Source	Use
197. Sacate Chino	<u>Hilaria cenchroides</u> H.B.K. (A.S. Hitchcock)	W508		Plateau west of Charcas	
198. Sacate Cochinillo	<u>Cenchrus pauciflorus</u> Benth. (A.S. Hitchcock)	W588		Charcas, near cornfield	
199. Sacate Cola Sorra	<u>Lycurus phleoides</u> H.B.K. (A.S. Hitchcock)	W592		Charcas mountain side	
200. Sacate Masarca	<u>Panicum obtusum</u> H.B.K. (A.S. Hitchcock)	W583		Charcas, near cultivated land	
201. Sacate Sevaidilla	<u>Sitanion</u> (Nutt.) J.G. Smith (A.S. Hitchcock)	W490		Charcas, protected hillside	
202. Sacaton	<u>Sporobolus Wrightii</u> Munro (AFW?)	W572		Charcas, enclosed hillside	
203. Salvia	unidentified	L5688 15140 L5688b	bundle of stems with leaves and flowers and pressed plant	Monterrey	Good for nourishing babies when mother cannot nurse. Boil in water and milk. Also for gas pain? Boil and drink.

204. Sanaparicio	unidentified	L5222 14960	bundles of stems with leaves and pressed	Charcas	For fevers
	Not recognized at U.S. National Museum	W919 14903	pressed branches with leaves, flowers	Charcas, San Diego	
205. Sangre de Grado	Not recognized at U.S. National Museum	W863 14878		Charcas plain	
206. San Nicolas	<u>Chrysactinia mexicana</u> Gray	L5260 14988	bundles of stems with leaves and flowers	Charcas	Chills (of women) when exposed. Taken as tea.
	<u>Chrysactinia mexicana</u> Gray	L5698 15150	bundles of whole plants	Monterrey	For women having babies. Taken with other herbs.
	<u>Chrysactinia mexicana</u> Gray	W598 14855	pressed, stem with leaves, flowers	Charcas, mountain top	
	<u>Menodora coulteri</u> Gray	W650 L5152 14862	pressed, whole plant	Charcas, enclosed hillside	

Spanish Name	Botanical Name	Catalog Number	Specimen	Location or Source	Use
207. San Rafael	unidentified	L5266 15004 L5266b	bundles of whole plants without roots pressed, whole plant	Charcas	Sweat bath and to prevent going to sleep after eating
208. Santa Isabel	unidentified	L5427 15042 L5427 15042	stems with leaves pressed, whole plant, no root	Charcas	Medicinal herb
	unidentified	L5697 15149 L5697 15149	bundle of stems with leaves pressed, whole plant	Monterrey	Medicinal herb
209. Santaura	unidentified	L5613 15064 L5613b	bundle of stems with leaves, flowers pressed	Monterrey	Medicinal herb
210. Saramado	unidentified	W651	no specimen	Charcas, enclosed hillside	A weed in corn fields
211. Saramago	*Brassica Eruca* L. *Eruca sativa*	W948 14918	mounted pressed whole plant	Charcas, near field of corn	

212. Sarsafras (Sasafras?)	unidentified	L5714 15167	pieces of bark		
213. Semillas Higeron	<u>Ricinus communis</u> L.	L5633 15084	beans	Monterrey	Laxative (castor oil bean)
214. Seniso	<u>Leucophyllum laevigatum</u> Standl.	L5265 15003	bundles of stems with leaves and flowers; pressed specimen	Charcas	Medicinal herb
	unidentified	L5644a 15095 L5644b	bundle of branches with leaves flowers; pressed specimen	Monterrey	Medicinal herb
215. Suelda	<u>Buddleia scordioides</u>	L5660 15112	bundles of stems with leaves, flowers	Monterrey	Medicinal herb
216. Tarumara or Tarumarra	<u>Asclepias setosa</u> Benth.	L5642 15093	roots	Monterrey	
	<u>Asclepias setosa</u> Benth.	15026	pieces of root	Charcas	
217. Tatalencho	<u>Selloa glutinosa</u> Spreng	L5232 14970	bundles of stems with leaves, flowers	Charcas	Rheumatism

Spanish Name	Botanical Name	Catalog Number	Specimen	Location or Source	Use
218. Te de Coral	*Bidens aurea* (Ait.) Sherrf (S. F. Blake)	W945 14915	mounted pressed whole plant without flower	Charcas, cornfield	Purge: Boil in water. Function like castor oil. One plant enough for one dose. Very effective laxative.
219. Te de la Hormiga	*Wedeliella glabra* (Choisy) Cockerell	L5213 14951	bundles of stems with leaves, flowers	Charcas	Kidney and bladder trouble: Boil with other herbs.
220. Te de Olor	unidentified	L5565 15054	bundles of stems with leaves; pressed specimen	Charcas	Purge: Boil in water.
221. Telempalcate	*Chaptalia seemanii* Hemsl.	L5571 15060	whole plants	Charcas	
222. Tianguis	unidentified	L5704b 15156	bundles of stems with leaves, flowers		

223. Tlachi-chinola or Tlanchi-chinole	unidentified	L5666 15118 L5273 15011	stems with leaves, flowers, also pressed stems, leaves, flowers	Monterrey	Medicine
224. Timbre or Timbe	Acacia fili-cioides	W1010 14927	no specimen	Charcas market	Pulque: to ferment
225. Tobaco Loco	Nicotiana tri-gonophylla Dunal	W502 14851	pressed, stem with leaves, flowers	Charcas, edge of barranca	Not for smoking
	Nicotiana tri-gonophylla Dunal	W578	no specimen	Charcas, old wall side of barranca	
226. Toluache	unidentified	W665	no specimen	Venado, edge of road	For excited animals: Leaves are used as with barba de chivo
227. Tomate de Campo	Physalis sordida Fern.	W802 14875	pressed, stem with leaves and part of flower	Charcas	
228. Tomillo	unidentified	W950 14920	no specimen	Charcas, mountain base	Stomach trouble

Spanish Name	Botanical Name	Catalog Number	Specimen	Location or Source	Use
	unidentified	L5628 15079	bundle of stems with leaves		
229. Torito	unidentified	W944 14914	mounted, stem with seedpods and whole plant	Charcas, broken ground	Lung (chest) trouble: Seeds are ground and drunk in water
230. Toronjil	unidentified	L5652a 15103	bundles of whole plants without roots and a pressed specimen	Monterrey	Medicinal herb
231. Trigillo Loco	<u>Avena</u> <u>fatua</u> L.	W510	no specimen	Charcas, roadside, inhabited area	
232. Tripa de Judas	<u>Parietaria</u> <u>pennsylvanica</u>	L5214 14952	peeled roots	Charcas	
233. Trompillo	<u>Solanum</u> <u>elaeagnifolium</u> Cav.	W570	no specimen	Charcas, enclosed hillside	To coagulate milk
	<u>Solanum</u> <u>elaeagnifolium</u> Cav. (C.V. Morton)	W905 14893	mounted stem with leaves, berries	Charcas, enclosed hillside	Eye trouble of goats or donkeys: Place 1, 2, or 3 seeds in eyes.

234. Tullidora	unidentified	L5695a L5695c 15147	branches with leaves, berries	Monterrey	
235. Venado (Lanten)	*Plantago major* L.	W638 14858	pressed, stem with leaves, seeds	Charcas	
	unidentified	L5623 15074 L5623b	bundle of stems with leaves, flowers; pressed specimen	Monterrey market	Fertility: Good for women who wish to have babies: Boil in water and drink.
236. Ventosidad	*Nama hispidum* Gray	L5683 15135	bundles of stems with leaves, flowers	Monterrey	Stomach trouble
	Nama palmeri Gray	W613 14856	collected specimen, root, leaves	Charcas, edge of cultivated field	Catarro: smell it (inhale)
	Nama undulatum H.B.K.	L5258 14996	bundles of stems with leaves	Charcas	Relief from gas pains.
	Nama undulatum H.B.K. (C.V. Morton)	W922 14906	mounted stems with leaves, flowers	Charcas, field	Cold: smell.

Spanish Name	Botanical Name	Catalog Number	Specimen	Location or Source	Use
237. Verbena (ocea de Lagayina)	?*Guazuma* sp. ?*Anazuma ulmifolia*	L5221 14959	bundles of whole plants without roots		
238. Verguensa (see Yerba de la Verguensa)					
239. Violeta	*Viola* sp.	L5615 15066	stems with flowers and leaves	Monterrey	Cough: Boiled with other herbs
240. Visvir-inda	*Castela texana*	W1086 14935	pieces of root	Charcas	
241. Wisachito	*Hoffmanseggia densiflora* Benth.	W562	no specimen	Charcas, enclosed hillside	
242. Yerba Blanca	not recognized at U.S. National Museum	W896 14885	mounted stem with leaves	Charcas, plateau near San Diego	Sores on back of horse: roots used. Leaves used for some kind of horse medicine, for bruises?
243. Yerba Blanco	unidentified	L5274 15012	pieces of root		Very poison-ous

244. Yerba Buena	unidentified	L5564 15053	bundles of stems with leaves, few flowers, also, pressed	Charcas	Good for women who have children and wish to congregate them. Colic: Boil in water and drink.
	unidentified	L5678 15130	bundles of stems with leaves and flowers, also, pressed	Monterrey	Digestion: Good for children.
245. Yerba del Buen Dia	Sida procumbens Sw.	L5271 15009	bundles of stems with leaves and flowers	Charcas	Boils
	Sida procumbens Sw.	L5669 15121	bundles of stems with leaves and flowers	Monterrey	Kidney trouble
	Sida procumbens Sw.	W866 14880	mounted, stems with leaves	Charcas, plain	
246. Yerba del Cancer	Acalypha lindheimeri Muell. Arg.	L5229 14967	bundles of whole plants without roots	Charcas	Medicinal herb

Spanish Name	Botanical Name	Catalog Number	Specimen	Location or Source	Use
	Acalypha hederaceae Torr.	L5653 14967	bundles of stems with leaves and flowers	Monterrey	Medicinal herb
247. Yerba Candelilla	*Pedilanthus pavanis*	L5703 15155	bundle of stems		
248. Yerba del Conejo (ocea de la amorana)	unidentified	L5268 15006	bundles of whole plants few roots		
249. Yerba del Gato	*Croton corymbulosus* Engelm.	W695 14868	pressed stems, leaves, flowers	Charcas, enclosed hillside	Susto: Boil in water
	unidentified	W868 14882	pressed stems, leaves, flowers	Charcas, plateau near San Diego	Piles. Boil in water and drink
	unidentified	W654	no specimen	Charcas, enclosed hillside	
	unidentified	L5211 14949	bundles of stems with leaves, flowers		

	unidentified	L5657 15109	bundles of whole plants		
250. Yerba del Golpe	<u>Gaura</u> <u>coccinea</u> Pursh	W901 14890	mounted, stems with leaves, flowers	Charcas, enclosed hillside	Bruises: leaves placed over bruised area
	<u>Gaura</u> <u>coccinea</u> Pursh	W653	no specimen	Charcas, enclosed hillside	Wounds and bruises: Boil in water and wash
	<u>Gaura</u> <u>coccinea</u> Nutt.	L5279 15017	bundles of stems with leaves, flowers	Charcas	
	<u>Gaura</u> <u>sinuata</u> Nutt.	L5658 15110	bundles of stems with leaves, seeds	Monterrey	
251. Yerba de la Hormiga	<u>Acalypha</u> <u>phleoides</u> Cav.	W640 14860	pressed stems with leaves and flowers	Charcas, enclosed hillside	
	<u>Wedeliella</u> <u>glabra</u> (Choisy) Cockerell	L5686 15138	bundles of stems with leaves flowers	Monterrey	Kidney trouble

Spanish Name	Botanical Name	Catalog Number	Specimen	Location or Source	Use
252. Yerba Jarrito	unidentified	W541	no specimen	Charcas, inhabited area	
253. Yerba Mora	_Solanum pterocaulon_ (_Solanum nigrum_)	W913 14897	no specimen	Charcas, enclosed hillside	Espanto (fright): Grind leaf and take juice of unripe fruit (?) Eruption of the blood: Rub the little pustule with the ripe fruit.
	Solanum pterocaulon Dun.	W643 14861	pressed stem, leaves, berries	Charcas, enclosed hillside	Inflammation of the skin: Use ripe (black) fruit.
	Solanum pterocaulon Dun.	L5432 15047	bundles of stems with leaves, berries	Charcas	Medicinal herb
	Solanum pterocaulon Dun.	L5698 15141	bundles of stems with leaves and some root	Monterrey	Medicinal herb
254. Yerba del Negrito	_Sphaeralcea hastatula_	W768	no specimen	Charcas, west of San Diego	

(Yerba Negrito)	Sphaeralcea angustifolia (Cav.) Don.	W557	no specimen	Charcas, enclosed hillside	
	Sphaeralcea angustifolia var. cuspidata Gray	W589	no specimen	Charcas, near cultivated land	
255. Yerba del Negro	Sphaeralcea angustifolia (Cav.) Don	L5661b 15113	bundles of whole plants without roots		
	Sphaeralcea hastulata Gray Not typical (Kearney)	W861 14876	mounted, pressed, stem with leaves, flowers	Charcas, plain	
256. Yerba Nis or Santa Maria or Operion	Tagetes florida Sweet	L5670 15122	bundles of stems with leaves, flowers	Monterrey	Medicinal herb
	Tagetes florida Sweet	L5267 15005	bundles of stems with leaves, flowers	Charcas	Sweat bath. Breakfast tea, boiled in water.
257. Yerba del Pajarito	unidentified	W642	no specimen	Charcas, enclosed hillside	
	unidentified	W815	no specimen	Aquila Mt. or Aguila?	

Spanish Name	Botanical Name	Catalog Number	Specimen	Location or Source	Use
258. Yerba del Pinacate	*Cassia Wislizeni* Gray	W728 L5439 14872	pressed branch with leaves, flowers	Charcas, plain shrub	
259. Yerba del Sapo	*Eryngium Wrightii* Gray	W923 14907	pressed stem with leaves and flowers	Charcas, arroyo near San Diego	Cough: Boil in water
	Eryngium Wrightii Gray	L5429 15044	bundles of whole plants	Charcas	Cough. Urine trouble
	unidentified	L5706 15159	bundles of stems with leaves and burrs	Monterrey	Medicinal herb
260. Yerba del Tomor	*Drymaria gracilis* C. and S. (C.V. Morton)	W916 14900	mounted stems with leaves, flowers	Charcas, San Diego	Tumor or swelling on hand or foot: Boil in water.
261. Yerba del Torito	unidentified	W737	no specimen	Bank of arroyo near water Charcas?	
262. Yerba del Venado	*Porophyllum filiforme* Rydb.	L5246 14984	bundles of stems with leaves, flowers	Charcas	Constipation

263. Yerba de la Verguensa	*Schrankia potosina* (Britt. and Rose) Standley	W899 14888	no specimen	Charcas, enclosed hillside	"plant of shame"
	Schrankia potosina (Britt. and Rose) Standley	W559	no specimen	Charcas, enclosed hillside	"plant of shame"
264. Yerba de la Virgen	unidentified	L5625 15076	bundle of stems with leaves, flowers also pressed	Monterrey	Medicinal herb
265. Yerba Vivora	*Calophanes linearis* Gray (*Dyschoriste linearis*)	L5680 15132	bundles of whole plants	Monterrey	Snakebite
266. Yerba de la Vivora	*Dyschoriste decumbens* (Gray) Kuntze	L5239 14977	bundles of whole plants	Charcas	Constipation: Boil in water and drink
267. Yerba Zorillo	*Chenopodium* sp.	L5663 15115	bundles of stems and flowers	Monterrey	Medicinal herb
268. Zacate Liso	*Muhlenbergia monticola* Buckl. (A.S. Hitchcock)	W618	no specimen	Charcas, edge of cornfield	

Spanish Name	Botanical Name	Catalog Number	Specimen	Location or Source	Use
269. Zarsa-parilla	*Krameria pauci-flora* DC.	L5231 14969	bundles of roots	Charcas	Blood, to purify and increase. Infected gums: used to clean.
	Krameria pauci-flora DC.	L5570 15059	roots, leaves	Charcas	Bad teeth
	Krameria pauci-flora DC.	L5712 15165	bundles of roots	Monterrey	Lack of blood: used with others.
270. Zarzafras	?*Elaphrin pubes-cens* Schl.?	L5710 15163	pieces of bark	Monterrey	

APPENDIX C

The Leslie A. White Collection
Albuquerque, 1941

In 1941 Leslie A. White, then a member of the faculty of the Department of Anthropology at the University of Michigan, purchased samples of dried medicinal herbs from B. Ruppe's drugstore in Albuquerque, New Mexico. These herbs were given to the Ethnobotanical Laboratory at the University of Michigan. The 23 items listed on the following pages apparently represent the druggist's entire inventory at the time of purchase. No information on usage was collected and several specimen are unidentifiable. Also, little is known about the clientele or sources of the herbs. However, it is important to note that this store was a source of medicinal herbs in 1941 in the Albuquerque area.

	Spanish Name	Botanical Name	Specimen
1.	Artemisia Yerba	Artemisia sp.	stems and leaves
2.	Caña Agria	Rumex hymenosepalus Torr.	sliced segments of roots
3.	Caña Fistula	Cassia sp.	seed pods
4.	Cañutillo	Ephedra sp.	stems
5.	Cáscara Nogal	Juglans sp.	bark
6.	Chia	Salvia sp.	seeds
7.	Contra Yerba	Kallstroemia californica (S. Wats.) Vail, var. brachystylis (Vail) Kearney & Peebles	sliced segments of roots
8.	Estafiate	Artemisia sp.	stems and leaves
9.	Flor Asar	Citrus sp.	flowers
10.	Flor de jamica	unidentified	dark flowers
11.	Hineldo	Anethum graveolens L. dill	seeds
12.	Oregano Mexicano	unidentified	stems and leaves
13.	Palo Brazil	Caesalpinia sp.	chips of wood
14.	Palo Mulato	unidentified	bark
15.	Pasmo	unidentified	stems and leaves
16.	Pasote	Chenopodium ambrosiodes L.	leaves
17.	Peonias	unidentified	roots
18.	Quassia	Quassia amara L.?	wood chips
19.	Yerba Anise	unidentified	stems and leaves
20.	Yerba Cancer	unidentified	stems
21.	Yerba Gobernadora	Larrea tridentata	stems and leaves

Spanish Name	Botanical Name	Specimen
22. Yerba Golondrina	Euphorbia sp.?	stems and leaves
23. Yerba Gordolobo	unidentified	stems and flowers

APPENDIX D

Juarez, Chihuahua, Market Collection, 1965

Karen C. and Richard I. Ford

In May, 1965, the Fords purchased herbs at the Mercado Cuauhtemoc for comparison with plants they were encountering in their work with Pueblo Indians in northern New Mexico. Samples of 38 herbs were purchased from the only herb vendor in this market--a man of 66 years who had been in the market since the late 1930's. His entire inventory consisted of over 150 herbs and other medicinal items, including patent medicines. This man obtained his herbs by collecting them himself as well as through purchases from other collectors. He had considerable knowledge of usages which were recorded for many of the items purchased. While a systematic study was not undertaken either with this collection or the Jones Collection (Appendix A) and the purposes for collecting the herbs were not the same, it is interesting to note the similarity of items available despite a gap of 33 years.

The herbs are listed on the following pages and are deposited in the Ethnobotanical Laboratory at the University of Michigan. Unfortunately, many items were in unidentifiable condition.

Spanish Name	Botanical Name	Catalog Number	Specimen	Use
1. Albaca	Ocimum Basilicum L. (sweet basil)	5317	leaves and stems	
2. Alfil-erillo	Erodium sp.	5318	whole plant	
3. Altamisa	Chrysanthemum parthenium ?	5319	flowers, leaves, and stems	
4. Babiza or Manzo	Anemopsis californica (Nutt.) Hook. and Arn.	5320	leaves, stems, and roots	For sores
5. Caballo	Equisetum sp.	5322	stems	Good for kidneys
6. Cachana	unidentified	5323	root	For woman after childbirth
7. Calco meca	unidentified	5324	bark	Tea
8. Caña Agua or Caña Agria	Rumex hymenosepalus Torr.	5325	root	To clean teeth
9. Canutillo	Ephedra sp.	5326	stems	Tea for stomach
10. Cenizo	Leucophyllum sp.?	5327	stems and leaves	
11. Collate	unidentified	5328	stems and leaves	Tea for stomachache

12. Copalquin	*Hintonia* sp.?	5329	bark	For stomach
13. Estafiate	*Artemisia* sp.	5330	leaves and stems	
14. Hediondilla Governadora	*Larrea tridentata* (DC.) Coville	5332	leaves and stems	For stomach
15. Hinojo	*Antheum graveolens* L. [dill]	5333	stems, umbells, and seeds	For a tea
16. Malva	*Malva* sp.?	5334	crumbled leaves and stems	For stomach
17. Manzanilla	*Matricaria* sp.?	5335	flowers, leaves and stems	Boil in water for tea for babies
18. Mejorana	*Origanum* sp.? [marjoram]	5336	leaves	Cooking herb
19. Orozuz	unidentified	5337	wood chips	For stomach
20. Osha or Chuchupate	*Ligusticum Porteri* Coult. and Rose	5338	root	
21. Pazote Comer	*Chenopodium* sp.	5339	leaves and stems	Cook with beans
22. Pazote de Sorillo	unidentified	5340	leaves and stems	Tea

Spanish Name	Botanical Name	Catalog Number	Specimen	Use
23. Poléo	unidentified	5341	leaves and stems	Take as sedative
24. Rosemary	*Rosmarinus officinalis* L.	5342	leaves and stems	
25. Ruda	*Ruta* sp.?	5343	leaves and stems	
26. Sabino Macho	unidentified	5344	leaves and stems	
27. Te	*Cymbopogon* sp.	5345	leaves	
28. Tomilla	*Thymus* sp. [thyme]	5346	leaves and stems	Cook with beans
29. Toronjil	*Cedronella mexicana* Benth.	5347	leaves and stems	For heart?
30. Valeriana	unidentified	5348	root	For headache: put herb water on head
31. Verbena	*Verbena* sp.?	5321	leaves and stems	For sores
32. Yerba Buena	*Mentha spicata* L.	5349	leaves and stems	
33. Yerba Cancer	unidentified	5350	leaves and stems	
34. Yerba Colorado	unidentified	5351	stems	Tea with milk and sugar

	or Chacota or Calderona			
35.	Yerba del Lobo	unidentified	5352	flowers, leaves, and stems	Take for cough
36.	Yerba de la Negrita	unidentified	5353	flowers, leaves, and stems	For sores and cuts
37.	Yerba del Sapo	unidentified	5354	stems and burrs	
38.	Yerba de la Vivora	unidentified	5355	leaves and stems	Boil in water, take for chills

APPENDIX E

Herb Collection

Theodore Roybal's Store, Santa Fe, New Mexico

The Roybal's store was founded in 1917 by Theodore Roybal and was housed for many years at the rear of 212, 214, 216 Galisteo Street in Santa Fe, New Mexico. In 1966 the store was owned and operated by a middle-aged couple, Hugo and Gloria Roybal Crowder at the above adress. As a "general" store it carried many items found in any grocery store: canned goods, packaged items, fresh meat, dairy products, and so on. In addition there were for sale knives and some camping equipment, household goods, cooking utensils, and specialty items such as taco molds and tortilla presses. A small yarn shop was housed separately. The store's inventory emphasized what the proprietors called "native goods" and "Mexican foods." The former included popular local foods such as chicos (boiled and sun-dried corn), red and green chile (fresh in season and dried), beans, blue cornmeal, white cornmeal, sprouted wheat flour, sun-dried apples, pinyon nuts, pozole (hominy), tortillas, and fresh greens such as quelites (lamb's quarters) and verdolagas (purslane). The "Mexican foods" included several types of chile peppers, black beans, chocolate, mole paste, piloncillo (raw sugar in cone form), and queso de tuna (prickly pear cactus candy).

Despite an extensive inventory of the above items, this store was perhaps most intriguing for its large collection of dried medicinal and cooking herbs displayed in small bins and neatly packaged and labeled in Spanish. To my knowledge no other store in northern New Mexico carried the number or variety of herbs available at this store. The herbs were arranged in alphabetical order and a list giving Spanish names and in some cases common English names for each herb was available to any customer. A number of non-plant items, such as piedra alumbre (alum stone), used medicinally were included.

Mrs. Crowder handled most of the incoming herbs and had some knowledge of usages but deferred to a Hispano employee when uncertain about a usage. Some of the herbs were stored in the basement prior to packaging and displaying for sale. Prices paid for herbs brought in locally varied with supply and demand, and herbs that did not sell were dropped from the inventory.

Several different sources were used for the procurement of the herbs. About half (65-70) were obtained locally. The proprietors themselves collected a few items, including hediondilla, oregano, and ruda, while an osha plant and several different mints were grown in a small garden behing the store. Most of the locally available herbs, however, were purchased from individuals who brought them in to sell. The suppliers were typically elderly Hispano men and women. Certain ones came several times each year with different seasonal herbs; others came once each summer and still others even less frequently. Only one woman delivered the herbs bagged and labeled according to use. In some cases individuals travelled considerable distances to bring herbs; suppliers came from at least as far away as Truchas and Vallecitos, New Mexico, the latter being more than fifty miles from Santa Fe. A few herbs were sold to the store by Indians. In the 1950's and 1960's Cochiti and Santo Domingo Indians supplied punche (tobacco) which they had raised. Occasionally younger people, sometimes Anglos, supplied herbs. During the mid-1960's a young Anglo was a regular supplier of a number of herbs. On one occasion he earned about $10.00 for barbasco, pague, romerillo, and alum stone which he brought in. He also tried to sell some caña agria, of which the store already had an abundant supply,and another herb which the store did not carry. He, as well as the other suppliers, did not indicate the source of his supply, and each collected his herbs independently.

Items not available locally were ordered from Mexico (42 altogether, including quasia, te de sena, caña fistula, and comino) or California (e.g. anís, alhucema, cascara de sagrada, asahar de naranjo), with one or two items being purchased from Texas or Colorado. A number of items were so popular that local supply often did not meet the demand, and the store ordered these items as necessary: inmortal, osha, romero, cachana, yerba de golpe, cardo santo, yerba de manso. A spice company in Texas supplied sassafras and a chemical company in Denver supplied piedralipe (copper sulfate). It is interesting to note the great distance travelled by a few of the items. The coral beads (important anti-evil eye charms) came from Italy; the very popular manzanilla was imported from Hungary via Mexico; and the non-local type of sangre de venado came from Malaysia via Mexico.

The clientele of the store was varied and included Hispanos, Indians, local Anglos, and tourists. Hispanos predominated and purchased the most herbs. Most lived, or had lived, in Santa Fe, though some came a considerable distance. The approximate area of utilization is bounded by the Taos area on the north, Las Vegas on the east, Jemez on the west, and Albuquerque on the south. Osha was the most popular item in the store. The less popular items were discontinued as supplies aged. Indians, especially from the nearby Rio Grande pueblos, were frequent customers, but purchased only a few items, particularly osha, chimaja, malvas, cilantro, and manzanilla. Anglos and tourists bought seasoning herbs, but, in a town with many tourist attractions, it is unlikely that very many tourists found their way to the store. Finally, mention should be made of the prices charged for the herbs. A small package containing a handful of an herb was generally priced under one dollar, but prices varied with supply and demand and a few items were priced much higher. Customers and other informants considered the prices somewhat high but for certain purchasers and for many of the items there was no alternative.

By 1969 the Crowders had sold the store and the building is now used for another business. A former employee of the Crowders continues (as of June 1974) to sell herbs in a smaller shop next door at 220 Galisteo Street.

In June 1971 Mr. Lujan's "Tienda de la Salud" had a thriving business in herbs in addition to a few other foodstuffs and cooking utensils. He retains the herb display cases of the old Roybal's Store and claims to sell more now than they ever did before. Still popular are alhucema, manzanilla, and osha and he mentioned that tilia, incienso, sassafras and mate were selling well. Perhaps the highlight of his tenure occurred recently when (in his words) a "hippie" from New York bought $76 worth of herbs at one time. Roybal's store may be gone, but the herb business continues to flourish on Galisteo Street in Santa Fe.

On the following charts are medicinal herb data collected by the author in 1966 in the Santa Fe and Española areas of New Mexico. With the exception of a very few items from published sources, only information obtained with reference to this collection is included. For further information on specific plants see the Glossary (Appendix F). It should be noted that mimeographed herb lists provided by the store were used to compile the charts. Some of the items listed were not available to me at the store but were obtained for study from the Museum of Navaho Ceremonial Art. A very few items listed were not available at all. Furthermore, several items sold by the store were and are apparently not in common use in northern New Mexico although they may be known to literate médicas through published sources. Finally, the condition of many herbs precluded positive identification. For those that were identifiable, the Latin names are derived from the books in the bibliography.

Here is a brief description of the informants used for this study.

1 = a middle-aged Hispano woman who had gathered medicinal data from relatives and friends, including several médicas, in the Santa Fe area.

2 = a middle-aged woman living near Española, who, though born in Mexico, has many local contacts.

3 = an elderly Hispano woman living near Española who has considerable first-hand knowledge of herbs and medicinal

practices in the area.

4 = a middle-aged Hispano woman, one of the proprietors of the store, who handled the purchasing of the herbs at the store.

4a = a middle-aged Hispano man who was an employee of the store in 1966. He was an herb dealer himself by 1969.

5 = a middle-aged Tewa man who has many Hispano contacts in the Española area.

(The information obtained from No. 3 is the most extensive.)

Spanish Name	Botanical Name [English Name]	Catalog Number	Specimen (part sold)	Source	Use
1. Ajenjibre	*Zingiber officinale* Roscoe [ginger]	no specimen	Dried root	Purchased from Mexico	Stomachache: add to coffee or water and drink (3). Fever: add to water for foot bath (1).
2. Ajonjoli	*Sesamum orientale* L. [sesame]	no specimen	Seeds	Purchased from Mexico	Cooking: an ingredient of mole sauce (1).
3. Albahaca; Alvacar	*Ocimum Basilicum* L. [sweet basil]	no specimen	Leaves	Purchased locally or from Mexico	Stomachache: add to coffee or water and drink (3). Charm: for good luck (1).
4. Albayalde	[white talc]	5238	White powder	Purchased locally or from Mexico	
5. Alcaparrosa	unidentified [zinc sulfate?]	5239	White powder	Purchased from Mexico	Asthma (4)
6. Alegría	*Amaranthus cruentus* L.	5240	Stems with leaves and seeds	Purchased locally	Heart trouble: grind with Azahar de Naranjo, Anís, cinnamon, Remolino, and deer's blood; add to wine and drink (3).

7.	Alfalfa, Semilla de	*Medicago sativa* L. [alfalfa seeds]	no specimen	Seeds	Purchased locally	Stomach pains (1)
8.	Alfilerillo	*Erodium cicutarium* L'Hér. [storksbill]	no specimen	Stems with leaves, flowers	Purchased locally	Urinary disorders: drink decoction (1)
9.	Alhucema	*Lavandula Spica* Cav. [lavender]	no specimen	Flowers	Purchased from California	Stomach gas (babies): give decoction to drink (1). Coughs: drink decoction (1).
10.	Alquitrán	unidentified	5356	Pieces resembling rocks	Purchased locally	Incense: burn (3)
*11.	Altamisa	*Chrysanthemum parthenium* (L.) Bernh.?	5241	Stems with leaves, flowers	Purchased locally	Stomachache: drink decoction (3). Colds: drink decoction (3).
	Altamisa de la Sierra	*Artemisia franserioides* Greene	no specimen	?	Purchased locally	Stomachache: chew leaves or drink decoction (3)
12.	Alumbre, Piedre	not a plant [alum stone]	no specimen	lumps of stone	Purchased locally	Teeth: grind into powder and use in a rinse to tighten teeth (1). Burns: apply to affected area (1).

* Asterisk refers to notes on page

Spanish Name	Botanical Name [English Name]	Catalog Number	Specimen (part sold)	Source	Use
13. Amole	*Yucca* sp.	no specimen	Root	Purchased locally	Cleansing: soap for washing hair and woolen clothing and blankets.
14. Amolillo	unidentified	no specimen	?	?	Not on latest list (6/66)
15. Añil del Muerto	*Verbesina enceli-oides* (Cav.) Benth.	5242	Stems, leaves, flowers	Purchased locally	Ulcers: boil flower in water and drink (3) (1). Flatulence: drink decoction. (Marquez, 1964)
16. Anís	*Pimpinella anisum* L. [anise]	no specimen	Seeds	Purchased from California	Colds: drink decoction to cause sweating and to break a cold (3). Baking: an ingredient in sweet rolls and Biscochitos (3). Heart trouble: see Alegría.
17. Anís Estrella	*Illicium verum* [star anise]	no specimen	Seed pods	Purchased from Mexico	Nerves and sleeplessness: drink decoction (1). Baking: use as Anís (1).

18.	Azafrán	Carthamus tinctorius L. [American saffron]	no specimen	Flowers	Purchased locally	Measles: give tea to babies "to help them break out" (1) (3). Fever: drink decoction (1) (3). Dye: for wool, yellow (3). Food coloring and spice: use in meatballs, chicken, soups, and bread pudding (1) (3).
19.	Azahar de Naranjo	Citrus sp. [orange flowers]	no specimen	Flowers	Purchased from California or Mexico	Most ailments: grind, drink in warm water (3). Heart trouble: see Alegria. Nerves: take tea to aid sleep (1) (2).
20.	Azucaroan; Piedra Azucar	not a plant [rock candy]	no specimen	Candy that looks like pebbles	?	Food: candy
21.	Azufre	not a plant [sulphur]	no specimen	Yellow powder	Purchased from Mexico or locally	Coughs: take as syrup mixed with molasses (1). Soils: apply powder (3). Suppositories: mix together with finely ground Punche, Manzanilla, Osha, Romerillo,

Spanish Name	Botanical Name [English Name]	Catalog Number	Specimen (part sold)	Source	Use
					Yerba Buena, Piloncillo, tar soap, and honey and roll into small cigar shapes (3). Most ailments: drink mixed with water (3).
22. Barba de Maiz	Zea mays [corn]	no specimen	Corn silk	Purchased locally	Urinary disorder: take as tea for diuretic (1). Witchcraft: witches use (3).
23. Barbasco	Croton texensis (Kl.) Muell. Arg.	5243	Leaves, flowers	Purchased locally	Rheumatism: grind dry leaves, mix with honey and rub on swollen areas (3)
24. Babiza	unidentified	no specimen	?	Formerly purchased from Mexico	Recently discontinued (6/66). Note: Babiza is an alternative name for Yerba Manza.
25. Borraja	Borago officinalis L.	5244	Leaves, flowers, stems	Purchased locally	Stomach ailments: drink tea (1). Bites or infections: apply with pork fat as poultice (1). Fever: drink tea (1) (2). Eye ailments: use strained tea as

						eyewash (1). Sleeplessness: drink tea (1).
26.	Brazíl	*Caesalpinia echinata*	5245	Pieces of wood	Purchased from Mexico	Heart trouble: add to wine and drink (3)
27.	Buena Senora	unidentified	no specimen	?	Formerly purchased from Mexico	Recently discontinued (6/66)
*28.	Cachana	unidentified	5323	Root, nubby	Purchased from Mexico	Charm: carry an unburned piece for protection from witches (3)
		Liatris sp?	5357	Root, smooth	Purchased locally	Charm: carry burned piece to protect against evil eye (1). Headache: burn and inhale (3) (1). Nosebleed: burn and inhale (1). Tonsilitis: grind and blow into tonsils to dry them up (1).
	Flor de Cachana	*Liatris* sp.		Whole plant, except root (not sold)	Given by a woman from Truchas, New Mexico	

	Spanish Name	Botanical Name [English Name]	Catalog Number	Specimen (part sold)	Source	Use
29.	Cadillos	Xanthium sp.	no specimen	Stems with burrs and leaves	Purchased locally	
30.	Cahania; Cañahuela; Cañuela	unidentified	5246	Stems, leaves	Purchased locally	
31.	Cal	not a plant [lime]	no specimen	?	Purchased locally	Cooking: use to make posole (3). Insecticide: put on plants (3).
32.	Calabaza, Semilla de	Cucurbita sp. [squash, pumpkin]	no	Seeds	Purchased from Mexico	Food: eat roasted (3)
33.	Calabazilla	Cucurbita foetidissima H.B.K. [wild gourd]	5247	Chunks of root	Purchased locally	Very poisonous (3)
34.	Caña Agria	Rumex hymenosepalus Torr.	5358	Sliced pieces of root	Purchased locally	Teeth: use as mouthwash to tighten teeth (1)
35.	Cañafistula	Cassia fistula L.	5248	Seed pods	Purchased from Mexico	
36.	Canela en Raja	Cinnamomum zeylanicum Breyn [stick cinnamon]	5249	Pieces of bark	Purchased from Mexico	Colds: drink as tea to cause sweating (1) Stomachache: add ground cinnamon and

						sugar to coffee or water and drink (3). Heart trouble: see Alegría. Canning: e.g. for preserved pears as flavoring (3).
37.	Canutillo; Popotillo	Ephedra sp.	5250	Stems with flowers	Purchased locally	Urinary disorders and venereal disease: drink as tea (1). Stomach disorders: drink as tea (3).
*38.	Cardo Santo	unidentified	5359	Leaves	Purchased locally or from Mexico	
39.	Cascara de Capulín	Prunus sp. [chokecherry]	no specimen	Pieces of bark	Purchased locally	
40.	Cascara de Encino	Quercus sp. [oak]	5251	Pieces of bark	Purchased locally	Sores, especially in mouth: apply (1)
41.	Cascara de granada	Punica Granatum L. [pomegranite]	no specimen	Pieces of peel	Scraped off unsold pomegranites at end of season	
42.	Cascara de Nogal	Juglans sp. [walnut]	no specimen	Pieces of bark	Purchased from California	Mouthwash (1)
43.	Cascara Sagrada	Rhamnus californica Esch. [California buckthorn]	5252	Small pieces of bark	Purchased from California	Laxative: drink as tea (1)

	Spanish Name	Botanical Name [English Name]	Catalog Number	Specimen (part sold)	Source	Use
44.	Cebadilla; Sebadilla	unidentified possibly *Swertia radiata* (Kellogg) Kuntze	5300	Piece of root	?	Recently discontinued (6/66)
45.	Cenizo	? *Leucophyllum* sp.	5253	Leaves	Purchased from Mexico	
46.	Chamizo Gediondo	*Artemisia tridentata* Nutt.	5254	Leaves	Purchased locally	
*47.	Chamiza, Yerba de; see also Yerba de Chamizo	? *Atriplex* sp.	5367 5308	Stems with leaves	Purchased locally	
48.	Chan	unidentified	5255	Leaves and stems	Purchased locally	Foreign particle in eye: place seed in eye to help remove particle (1)
49.	Chimja	*Cymopterus purpureus* S. Wats.	no specimen	Leaves	Purchased locally	Popular with Indians as well as Spanish-Americans (4). Stomachache: chew leaves (3). Food: raw roots; use leaves to flavor beans or peas (3).

50.	Cilantro; Culantro	Coriandrum sativum L. [coriander]	no specimen	Seeds	Purchased locally	Popular with Indians as well as Spanish-Americans (4). Sedative: drink tea (1). Cooking: use fresh leaves in soup; seeds in tamales and carne adovado (3).
51.	Clavo Entero	*Caryophyllus aromaticus* [whole cloves]	no specimen	Dried flower buds	Purchased from Mexico	Cooking and baking: flavoring spice (5). Toothache: hold in mouth (5).
52.	Cola de Caballo	*Equisetum* sp.	no specimen	Stems	Purchased locally	
53.	Comino	*Cuminum odorum* [cumin]	no specimen	Seeds	Purchased from Mexico	Cooking: flavoring, add to red chile sauce (3)
54.	Contrayerba	*Kallstroemia californica* (Wats.) Vail var. *brachystylis* (Vail) Kearney and Peebles	5256	Peeled roots	Purchased locally	Tic: grind, sift, and rub externally on affected areas (3)
55.	Copalquín	*Hintonia* sp. *Coutarea* sp.	no specimen	pieces of bark	Purchased from Mexico	
56.	Corales	not a plant [red-orange sea coral]	no specimen	Small cut beads	Purchased from Italy	Evil eye charm: babies wear bracelets of coral beads to protect

	Spanish Name	Botanical Name [English Name]	Catalog Number	Specimen (part sold)	Source	Use
						against evil eye (3)
57.	Coral Prepardo	not a plant [powdered sea coral]	5257	Fine powder	Purchased from Mexico	Heart trouble: mix with deer's blood, gold leaf, and wine; drink as needed (1)
58.	Coronillo	unidentified no specimen available	no specimen	?	?	Not on latest list (6/66), perhaps discontinued
59.	Costomate	unidentified	5258	Pieces of stem	Purchased from Mexico	Soon to be discontinued (6/66); doesn't sell
60.	Cota	_Thelesperma_ sp.	no specimen	Stems with leaves and flowers	Purchased locally	Beverage: drink as tea
61.	Damiana	unidentified	5259	Stems with leaves and flowers	Purchased locally	
62.	Escoba de la Vívora; Yerba de la Vívora; Collálle	_Gutierrezia Sarothrae_ (Pursh) Britt. and Rusby	no specimen	Stems, flowers	Purchased locally	Rheumatism: mix with Yerba de Caballo (not in this collection; ? _Senecio_ sp.) and water to make a bath (3). Menstrual cramping and diarrhea, especially after childbirth:

						take as tea with Yerba Buena and Estafiate. (Marquez, 1964)
63.	Estafiate; Ajenjo	Artemisia sp.	5260	Stems with leaves, flowers	Purchased locally	Stomachache: drink as tea (3). Menstrual cramping and diarrhea: see Escoba de la Vívora.
64.	Goma de Trementina	unidentified [? pine gum]	5261	Lumps of various size	Purchased locally	
65.	Hediondilla Governadora	Larrea tridentata (DC.) Coville [creosote bush]	no specimen	Stems with leaves	Collected by store keepers in southern New Mexico	Swelling and rheumatism: grind and wrap with cloth around affected area (3)
66.	Hinojo	Foeniculum vulgare [fennel]	5262	Stems with umbells, seeds, leaves	Purchased locally	Cooking herb
67.	Hojase	unidentified possibly Flourensia cernua DC. [Hoja sen]	5263	Leaves	Purchased from Mexico	
68.	Incienso	unidentified possibly from Encelia farinosa	5360	Small pebblelike lumps	Purchased from Mexico	Incense: burn (3)
69.	Inmortal	Asclepias capricornu Woodson	5264	Large pieces of root	Purchased locally or from Mexico (the latter may be	Cuts: grind and apply (4). Nosebleed: grind and inhale (3).

Spanish Name	Botanical Name [English Name]	Catalog Number	Specimen (part sold)	Source	Use
				different species)	Head cold: grind and place on nose with salt to cause sneezing (3). Internal bruises: drink as tea (3).
70. Laurel, Hojas de	unidentified possibly <u>Litsea</u> sp.	no specimen	Leaves	Purchased from California	
71. Linaza	<u>Linum</u> sp. [flax]	no specimen	Seeds	Purchased from Mexico	Ulcers (4). Wave set for hair (4).
72. Lúpulo	? <u>Humulus</u> <u>Lupulus</u> [hops]	5265	Flowers	Purchased from Mexico	
73. Malvas	<u>Malva</u> sp.	5266	Stems with leaves and flowers	Purchased locally	Popular with Indians as well as Spanish-Americans (4). Hemorrhaging (gynecological): drink as tea with raisins added (3).
74. Manzanilla	<u>Matricaria</u> sp. [Chamomile]	no specimen	Stems with leaves and flowers	Purchased from Mexico, imported from Hungary	Popular with Indians as we;; as Spanish-Americans (4). Stomachache: drink as tea (3). Colds: drink as tea (3). Beverage for babies:

						give sweetened tea (3) Suppositories: see Azufre.
75.	Maravilla, Flor de	unidentified	5267	Flowers	Purchased locally	
76.	Maravilla, Raiz de	? *Mirabilis multiflora* (Torr.) Gray [wild 4 o'clock]	5268	Large pieces of root	Purchased locally	Rheumatism: grind root into powder and rub on affected areas (3)
77.	Mariola	*Artemisia* sp.	5269	Stems with leaves and flowers	Purchased locally	
78.	Mastranzo; Mostranzo	*Marrubium vulgare* [horehound]	5361	Stems with leaves and flowers	Purchased locally	Boils and other external infections: boil in water and apply (3)
79.	Maza	no specimen available; probably *Myristica* sp. [mace]	no specimen	?	Purchased from Mexico	Recently discontinued (6/66)
80.	Mejorana	no specimen available; probably *Origanum* sp. [sweet marjoram]	no specimen	? Leaves, probably	Purchased from Mexico	Cooking herb
81.	Menta	unidentified possibly *Mentha arvensis*	5270	Stems with leaves	Purchased locally	

Spanish Name	Botanical Name [English Name]	Catalog Number	Specimen (part sold)	Source	Use
82. Mostaza, Semilla de	*Brassica* sp. [mustard seed]	no specimen	Seeds	Purchased from Mexico	Stomachache: place seeds in cold water and drink (3)
83. Naranjo, Hojas de	*Citrus* sp. [orange leaves]	no specimen	Leaves	Purchased from California or Mexico	
84. Nebada	*Nepeta* sp. [catnip]	5271	Leaves, flowers, and seeds	Purchased from Mexico	For cats
85. Nebrina	? *Juniperus* sp.	no specimen	Berries	Purchased from California	
86. Nogal, Hojas de	? *Juglans* sp. [walnut leaves]	no specimen	Leaves	?	
87. Nuez Entera Moscada	*Myristica* sp. [nutmeg]	no specimen	Whole nutmegs	Purchased from Mexico	Stomach ailments: powder and add to coffee and drink (5). Headache: grind and place on head (3). Paralysis, one side of face: apply plaster of honey, Punche, cinnamon, and nutmeg; also, dab on cotton and place in ear (3).

88.	Oregano	Monarda menthaefolia Graham [horsemint]	5272	Stems with leaves and flowers	Purchased locally or gathered by storekeepers	Coughs: drink as tea (3). Cooking herb (3).
*89.	Oreja de Raton	unidentified	5273a; 5273b 5273c	Stem with leaves Stems with leaves and flowers Stems with leaves and flowers	Purchased locally	
90.	Oro Volador	not a plant [gold leaf]	no specimen	Small pieces of gold leaf	Purchased from an art shop	Heart trouble: mix with deer's blood and drink as needed (4)
91.	Oshá	Ligusticum Porteri Coult. and Rose	5274	Large pieces of root	Purchased locally or from Mexico	Most popular item in collection with both Indians and Spanish-Americans (4). Cuts: grind and apply (3). Stomach ailments: che chew root (3). Snakes (charm): carry a piece to keep them away (3). Suppositories: see Azufre

Spanish Name	Botanical Name [English Name]	Catalog Number	Specimen (part sold)	Source	Use
92. Pagué	unidentified probably <u>Dyssodia papposa</u> (Vent.) Hitchc.	5275	Stems with leaves and flowers	Purchased locally	Diarrhea: boil flowers in water and drink (3). Stomachache: take as tea (1).
93. Palo Amargo; Palo Crozuz; Palo Amar-illo	unidentified	5276	Chips of wood	Purchased from Mexico	
94. Palo Mediono	unidentified	5277	Stems and leaves	?	Does not appear on either list prepared by the store
95. Parraco	no specimen available	no specimen	?	?	Recently discontinued (6/66)
96. Pazote; Epazote	<u>Chenopodium ambrosioides</u> L.	5278	Flowers and leaves	Purchased locally	Stomachache: chew dried leaves (3). Cooking: add to beans for flavor (3).
*97. Perejil	unidentified possibly <u>Petroselinum crispum</u> [parsley]	5279	Leaves and stems	Purchased in winter from Mexico	Cooking herb
98. Pescado, Raiz de	unidentified	5280	Small pieces of root	Purchased from Mexico	

99.	Piedralipe; Piedra Azul	not a plant [copper sulfate]	5281	Lumps of blue minaral	Purchased from a chemical company in Colorado	Agriculture: use to treat wheat seed and corn seed before planting (3)
100.	Pimienta Entera	_Piper nigrum_ L. [black pepper]	no specimen	White peppercorns	Purchased from Mexico or from a spice company in Texas	Coughs: take with warm water (3). Stomachache: take with warm water (3). Cooking: use for seasoning (3).
101.	Pionilla	unidentified	5282	Roots	Pruchased from Mexico	
102.	Plumajillo	_Achillea lanulosa_ Nutt.	5283	Stems and leaves	Purchased locally	Stomach ailments: drink as tea (1) (3)
103.	Polellito Chino	unidentified possibly _Hedeoma oblongifolia_	5284	Stems, leaves and flowers	Purchased locally	
104.	Poléo	_Hedeoma nanum_ Torr.	5362	Stems and leaves	Purchased locally	Fever: drink as tea (3)
105.	Popotillo; Canutillo	_Ephedra_ sp.	5285a; 5285b; 5250	Stems	Purchased locally	See Canutillo
106.	Prodigiosa	unidentified	5286	Stems, leaves and flowers	Purchased from Mexico	
107.	Punche	_Nicotiana rustica_ [tobacco]	5287	Leaves	Purchased locally from	Earache: roll leaves with Ruda to form a

Spanish Name	Botanical Name [English Name]	Catalog Number	Specimen (part sold)	Source	Use
				Keresan Indians	cigar; light and blow smoke into ear (3). Tick in ear: boil, dab on cotton, place in ear; tick will come out (3). Suppositories: see Azufre.
108. Quasia; Cuasia	? Quassia amara L.	5288	Wood chips	Purchased from Mexico	
*109. Quelites	Chenopodium sp. [lamb's quarters]	5289	Leaves	Purchased locally	Food: cook with chile, onion, and bacon (3)
110. Raiz del Indio	unidentified	5290	Pieces of root	Purchased locally or from Mexico	
111. Raiz del Lobo; Yerba del Lobo	Helenium Hoopesii Gray	5291	Roots	Purchased locally or from Mexico (the latter may be a different species)	Internal bruises: grind and drink with water (3). Constipation: grind, mix with brandy or whiskey and drink. (Van der Eerden, 1948)
112. Raiz del Oso; Yerba del Oso	unidentified possibly Heracleum lanatum	5363	Chunks of root	Purchased locally or from Mexico	

113. Raiz de Sangre; see Yerba de Sangre	no specimen available unidentified	no specimen	?	?	
*114. Remolino	not a plant [resin-like deposit from bees]	no specimen	Small pebbles and resin from bees	Purchased locally	Removed from store list because it is hard to obtain. Demand always far greater than the supply. Heart trouble: see Alegría.
115. Romero	<u>Rosmarinus officinalis</u> L. [rosemary]	no specimen	Leaves	Purchased from Mexico or locally on occasion	Colds: boil in water and drink (3). Post-partal hemorrhage: use with heated bricks to fumigate. (Marquez, 1964)
116. Romerillo	<u>Artemisia</u> ?<u>filifolia</u> Torr.	5292	Stems with leaves and flowers	Purchased locally	Stomach ailments: grind into powder, boil and drink (3). Suppositories: see Azufre.
117. Rosa de Castilla	<u>Rosa</u> sp. [wild rose]	no specimen	Flowers	Purchased locally (yellow) or from Mexico (pink)	Fever: drink as tea (3). Sore throats and fever blisters: hold in mouth (3).
118. Rosatilla; Rositilla	unidentified	5293	Stems, leaves	?	Not on most recent list (6/66)

Spanish Name	Botanical Name [English Name]	Catalog Number	Specimen (part sold)	Source	Use
119. Ruda	*Ruta* sp.	5364	Leaves	Purchased locally; gathered by the storekeepers locally; or purchased from Mexico	Earache: roll leaves with punche to form cigar; light and blow smoke into ear (3)
120. Sabino Macho	*Juniperus communis* L. or *Juniperus sibirica* Burgsd. [dwarf juniper]	5365	Branch portion with needles	Purchased locally	Urinary disorders: drink tea made from needles (3)
121. Sagui; Sagu	unidentified	5294	Leaves	Purchased from Mexico	
122. Salvia	unidentified possibly *Salvia* sp. or *Hyptis* sp.	5295	Leaves	Purchased from Mexico	
*123. Sangre de Venado	not a plant [deer's blood or dragon's blood]	no specimen	Dried flakes of blood or a substance resembling blood	Purchased locally or from Mexico which imports it from Malaysia	Popular and expensive. Heart trouble: add with gold leaf to wine and drink as needed (4). Heart trouble: grind with Alegría, Azahar, Anís, cinnamon, Remolino; add wine and drink (3).

124. Sanguinaria	unidentified	5296	Stems and roots with a few leaves	Purchased from Mexico or locally on occasion	
125. Santa Rita	unidentified	5297	Stems, leaves, flowers	?	Not on most recent list (6/66). Discontinued?
126. Sarza; Zarza	unidentified possibly _Rubus_ sp.	5298	Flower petals	Purchased from Mexico	
127. Sasafras	_Sassafras_ sp.	no specimen	Bark of roots	Purchased from Mexico or a spice company in Texas	Tonic: good for blood; drink as tea (1)
128. Saúco, Flor	_Sambucus mexicana_ Presl	5299	Flowers with seeds	Purchased from Mexico	
129. Sebadilla see Cebadilla					
130. Tamarindo	_Tamarindus indica_ L.	no specimen	Dried fruit--bean pods	Purchased from Mexico	
131. Te de Sena	unidentified possibly _Cassia_ sp. [Senna leaves]	no specimen	Leaves	Purchased from Mexico	Laxative: boil and drink (3)
132. Tequesquite	not a plant [crude sodium bicarbonate]	5301	Lumps of rock	Purchased locally	Baking: e.g. in puchas (a type of cookie) (3)

Spanish Name	Botanical Name [English Name]	Catalog Number	Specimen (part sold)	Source	Use
133. Tomillo	unidentified possibly Thymus sp. [thyme?]	5366	Leaves	Purchased from Mexico	
134. Toronjil	? Cedronella mexicana Benth.	5302	Pieces of stem	Purchased from Mexico	
135. Trabul	no specimen available unidentified	no specimen	?	?	Recently discontinued (6/66)
136. Tranze	unidentified	5303	Stems, leaves, flowers (a few)	Purchased from Mexico or locally on occasion	Doesn't sell; soon to be discontinued (6/66)
137. Tronadora	unidentified	5304	Stems and some seeds	Purchased from Mexico	
138. Ventosidad	? Nama sp.	5305	Stems, leaves and flowers	Purchased from Mexico or locally	
139. Verbena	Verbena sp.	no specimen	Stems with a few leaves, flowers	Purchased from Mexico or locally	Stomach ailments: drink as tea (3)
140. Yerba Buena	Mentha spicata L.	no specimen	Leaves	Purchased locally or from Mexico when necessary	Stomachache: drink as tea (3). Suppositories: see Azufre.

						Menstrual cramping and diarrhea: see Escoba de la Vívora.
141.	Yerba del Buey	? Grindelia aphanactis Rydb.	5306	Stems, leaves and flowers	Purchased locally	
142.	Yerba Cancer	unidentified	5307	Stems, leaves	Purchased from Mexico	
143.	Yerba de Chamizo see also Chamiza, Yerba de	? Atriplex sp.	5308 5367	Stems and leaves	?	Not on either list prepared by the store under this name
144.	Yerba de la Golondrina	Euphorbia sp.	no specimen	Leaves and stems	Purchased locally or from Mexico	
145.	Yerba del Golpe	unidentified possibly Gaura sp. or Oenothera sp.	5309	Stems with leaves	Purchased locally or from Mexico	
146.	Yerba del Lobo see Raiz del Lobo	Helenium Hoopesii Gray				
147.	Yerba del Manzo; Yerba Manza	Anemopsis californica (Nutt.) Hook. and Arn.	5310	Stems	Purchased locally or from Mexico on	Diarrhea: drink as tea (1). Boils: use infusion

Spanish Name	Botanical Name [English Name]	Catalog Number	Specimen (part sold)	Source	Use
				occasion	as wash. (Jones, 1932)
148. Yerba Mate	? <u>Ilex</u> sp.	5311	Leaves	Purchased from Mexico	
149. Yerba de la Negrita	<u>Sphaeralcea</u> sp.	5312	Stems with leaves and flowers	Purchased locally	Hair rinse (1)
150. Yerbaniz	unidentified possibly <u>Tagetes</u> sp.	5313	Stems and leaves	Purchased locally or from Mexico	
151. Yerba del Oso see Raiz del Oso					
152. Yerba de Sangre	<u>Berberis</u> <u>repens</u>	5368	Leaves	Purchased locally or from Mexico	
153. Yerba Santa	? <u>Eriodictyon</u> <u>agustifolium</u> Nutt.	5314	Leaves and flower parts	Purchased locally or from Mexico	
*154. Yerba del Sapo	unidentified possibly <u>Franseria</u> sp. or <u>Eryngium</u> sp.	5315a	Stems and burrs	Purchased locally or from Mexico	Rheumatism: grind and apply externally (3)
		5315b	Stems and flowers		

155. Yerba de la Vivora see Escoba de la Vivora					
156. Zacate Límon; Té Límon	*Cymbopogon citratus*	no specimen	Leaves	Purchased from Mexico	Beverage: drink as tea
157. Zarzaparilla	unidentified possibly *Smilax* sp.; *Humulus americanus*; or *Krameria* sp.	5369	Stems and roots	Purchased from Mexico	Tonic: take as tea, good for blood (1)
*158. Zuelda de Zuelda	unidentified	5316a	Stems and leaves	Purchased from Mexico	Broken bones: use to make casts (1)
		5316b	Stems with thorns and leaves		

NOTES IDENTIFIED WITH A (*) ON THE CHARTS

11. Altamisa. The information given by informants was inconsistent. Often this term is used to refer to either of the two different plants noted. The Artemisia grows wild locally while the Chrysanthemum would grow locally only if planted. The latter is similar to Manzanilla. The former resembles Tansy (Tanacetum vulgare) which is confused with it by some individuals and used similarly.

28. Cachana. Published works consulted do not suggest which plant (or plants) is the source of this very commonly used root. A flower (Flor de Cachana) was identified by V.H. Jones and R.I. Ford as Liatris sp., but no sample of root accompanied this flower. From the numerous different specimens of Cachana shown to me by informants I can only suggest that there may be more than one plant in northern New Mexico.

38. Cardo Santo. This name refers to several different plants in northern New Mexico and Mexico, and the uses vary. A positive identification of the specimen was not possible, and it is likely that the store may purchase different plants under this name on different occasions.

47. Chamiza, Chamizo, and Chamisa. Various published sources and various informants seem to confuse these terms. The first two names usually refer to Atriplex except when another word is added, such as Gediondo (#46.). The third name is usually for Chrysothamnus nauseosus (rabbit-brush).

89. Oreja de Raton. Positive identification was not possible. The three different samples were not all from the same plant. Different plants were undoubtedly sold to the store on different occasions under the same name.

97. Perejil. My best informants did not know this term as a name for parsley.

109. Quelites. Several species of Amaranthus are also known by this name. The term is used in much the same way as "greens" is used in certain American (English) dialects.

114. Remolino. The term literally means "whirlwind." This substance is used by San Juan Indians to treat "windstrike" which usually includes among its symptoms partial facial paralysis. This condition is thought to be caused by a whirlwind.

115. Sangre de Venado. The imported type is probably "Dragon's Blood," a substance from a type of palm tree. The locally pur-

chased type is apparently actual dried blood from a deer.

154. *Yerba del Sapo*. Positive identification was not possible. Several different plants are known by this name in the Southwest and in Mexico. Again, different plants are probably purchased by the store at different times under the same name.

158. *Zuelda de Zuelda*. Two different plants were being sold at the same time under this name. Neither was identifiable.

APPENDIX F

A GLOSSARY OF SPANISH-NAMED MEDICINAL PLANTS

This glossary brings together a considerable amount of medicinal herb data from many different sources both published and unpublished. It has grown from my interest in Hispano medicinal practices in northern New Mexico. Many plants used by New Mexican Hispanos, as well as by certain Pueblo Indian groups, are widely used in Mexico and in areas of the southwestern United States. Also, a particular Spanish name may apply to several different plants in different geographical areas. Most botanical reference books provide few local Spanish names, and ethnographic works often are incomplete with respect to either the Spanish name or the botanical identifications. Thus, it seemed appropriate to collate what appeared to be the best published ethnobotanical data, together with several unpublished bodies of data, including my own field notes, principally from the summer of 1966.

The data in Appendices A-E are included in the glossary. All of these collections, including my own field collections, are deposited at the Ethnobotanical Laboratory at the University of Michigan. In addition, mention should be made of the inclusion of information from the unpublished manuscripts by Riley and Trujillo (1956), and Schulman and Smith (1962). All sources used to compile the glossary are included in the bibliography.

The supplement includes plants for which a Spanish name was lacking but other information was available in the literature and collections consulted.

Informants for data gathered by me are as follows:

1 = a middle-aged Hispano woman who has gathered medicinal data from relatives and friends, including several médicas, in the Santa Fe area.

1a = an elderly Hispano woman, mother of #1.

2 = a middle-aged woman living near Española, who, though born in Mexico, has many local contacts.

3 = an elderly Hispano woman living near Española who has considerable first-hand knowledge of herbs and medicinal practices in the area. She provided the greatest quantity of information.

4 = a middle-aged Hispano woman, one of the proprietors of Roybal's Store (see also Appendix E) in Santa Fe during the early 1960s, who handled the purchasing of the herbs at the store.

4a = a middle-aged Hispano man who was an employee of Roybal's Store in 1966. A knowledgable herb dealer, he had his own store by 1969.

5 = a middle-aged Tewa Indian man who has many Hispano contacts in the Española area.
6 = a late middle-aged mestizo, born in Zacatecas, living in Mexico City in 1966.
7 = a middle-aged Tewa woman, married to a Hispano, living with her elderly Tewa grandmother, who was bilingual (Tewa and Spanish) and knowledgeable in local plant lore, Hispanic as well as Tewa.
8 = a late middle-aged vendor of herbs at the Juarez Market in 1965.

Spanish Name	Botanical Name	Location	Reference	Use
1. Aceite Linas	not a plant -- linseed oil?	New Mexico-Spanish	Shulman and Smith, 1962	Rheumatic pains: apply to affected area and cover with leaves of wild tobacco and warm cloths
2. Aceite de Olivo	not a plant -- olive oil	New Mexico-Spanish	Shulman and Smith, 1962	Massage: "it calms the nerves" use with pine pitch. Earache: use with cloves.
3. Aceite Quemado	not a plant -- burnt sugar and kerosene	New Mexico-Spanish	Shulman and Smith, 1962	Croup
4. Aceitilla	_Bidens leucantha_ (L.) Willd.	Valley of Mexico-Tepotzlan	Redfield, 1928 Field, 1953	Eye trouble: (caused in a baby by the approach of an individual who has recently had sexual intercourse) boil with raisins, Sauca (_Sambucus mexicana_ Presl.), and umbilical cords
	unidentified	Durango-Durango	Riley and Trujillo, 1956	Kidney troubles and cloudy urine: mix with Manzanilla (_Malvaviscus_) and cornsilk and boil, drink at night

Spanish Name	Botanical Name	Location	Reference	Use
	unidentified	Durango-La Ferreria	Riley and Trujillo, 1956	Kidney trouble: boil dry stems and leaves, leave overnight, drink as needed for next 9 days
	unidentified	Durango-San Pedro (across river from La Ferreria)	Riley and Trujillo, 1956	Kidney troubles: boil fresh or dry leaves and take liquid each night as needed
5. Acetilla	Bidens bigelovii	Chihuahua-Tarahumar	Pennington, 1963b	Food: boil, drain and fry leaves or add to beans
6. Aguacate	Persea americana	Chihuahua-Tepehuán	Pennington, 1963a	Diarrhea: crush seeds of mature fruits and make tea. Aching gums: place crushed seeds between cheek and gums. Goiter: apply poultice. Wounds and inflammation: apply pulp of mature fruit.
7. Aguapá	Typha latifolia L.	New Mexico-Spanish	Curtin, 1947	Pillows: use for stuffing Baskets: weave leaves
8. Agenjo	Artemisia mexicana Willd.	New Mexico-Spanish	Curtin, 1947	See Estafiate

(Ajenjo)	Artemisia vulgaris	Valley of Mexico-Tepepan	Madsen, 1965	Anger sickness: make tea with other "hot" herbs (e.g., anise, Cedrón) if person so afflicted has also eaten mushrooms
9. Agrito	Oxalis albicans H.B.K.	San Luís Potosí-Charcas	Whiting, 1934	
	Oxalis leonis Knuth	San Luís Potosí-Charcas	Whiting, 1934	
	Pellaea cordata (Cav.) J. Sm.	San Luís Potosí-Charcas	Whiting, 1934	
10. Ajenjibre	Zingiber officinale Roscoe	New Mexico-Spanish	Ford, 1966	Stomachache: add to coffee or water and drink (3). Fever: add to water for foot bath (1).
	Zingiber officinale Roscoe	New Mexico-Spanish	Van Der Eerden, 1948	Stomach trouble and fever: apply plaster of ginger and Punche (Nicotiana) to soles of feet overnight
11. Ajo	Allium sativum L.	New Mexico-Spanish	Curtin, 1947	Diphtheria: as preventative, wear around neck. Toothache: crush clove of garlic against gum. Earache: place on lamb's wool with salt and place in ear. Flatulence: roast, clean, chew and swallow with cold water.

Spanish Name	Botanical Name	Location	Reference	Use
				Snakebite: apply poultice of fresh mashed plant. Charm to rid girl of suitor: place at cross-roads.
		New Mexico-Spanish	Shulman and Smith, 1962	High blood pressure: roast and use internally. Asthma: externally. Pus: use to draw out and place in bandage of wound to ward off infection.
12. Ajonjoli	_Sesamum_ _indicum_ L.	New Mexico-Spanish	Ford, 1966	Food: an ingredient of mole sauce (1).
13. Alamillo	_Populus_ _tremuloides_	Chihuahua-Tepehuán	Pennington, 1963a	Menstrual pains, to stimulate parturition, and/or as tonic after parturition: make tea with bark
14. Álamo	_Populus_ _tremuloides_	Chihuahua-Tarahumar	Pennington, 1963b	Parturition: take decoction to stimulate birth
	Populus _fremontii_ Wats.	Baja California-Paipai	Owen, 1963	Bruises, aching joints, wounds: apply heated leaves
15. Álamo Blanco, Corteza de	_Populus_ sp.	San Luís Potosí-Charcas	Lundell, 1934	

16. Álamo de Hoja Redonda	_Populus wislizeni_ Wats.	New Mexico-Spanish	Curtin, 1947	Boils: make poultice of ashes of burned bark, cornmeal and water. Dropsy: take decoction of leaves. Broken bones: simmer bark to make thick syrup to apply as cast. Food: eat young pods of female tree raw.
17. Álamo Sauco	_Populus angustifolia_ James	New Mexico-Spanish	Curtin, 1947	Swollen gums or ulcerated tooth: dip cotton in cold water and apply to affected area
		New Mexico-Spanish	Shulman and Smith, 1962	Fever: tea from flower; tea from bark. Sweat baths: bark used.
18. Albáca; Albahaca	_Ocimum basilicum_ L.	New Mexico-Spanish	Curtin, 1947	Menstrual and labor pains: tea. Diarrhea: tea with sugar and nutmeg. Emmenagogue: eat a pinch, drink water. Earache: grind leaves, add oil and place drops in ear. Appetite (to increase): boil and take as tea. Colic: give sweetened tea to babies. Charm: for good luck and to correct wayward husband.

Spanish Name	Botanical Name	Location	Reference	Use
		New Mexico-Spanish	Shulman and Smith, 1962	Stomachache: tea. Aire: grind up with coriander, cinnamon, anise and nuts and rub on face while sweating.
(Alvacar)	_Ocimum_ _basilicum_ L.	New Mexico-Spanish	Van Der Eerdon, 1948	Parturition (to hasten): make tea
	Ocimum _basilicum_ L.	New Mexico-Spanish	Ford, 1966	Stomachache: add to coffee or water and drink (3)
(Albaca)	_Ocimum_ _basilicum_ L.	Chihuahua-Juarez	Ford and Ford, 1965	
(Albahaca)	_Ocimum_ _micranthum_ Willd.	Valley of Mexico-Tepotzlan	Redfield, 1928	Earache: place small amount in ear
	Ocimum _basilicum_ L.	Coahuila-Torreón	Kelly, 1965	Stomachache: drink decoction. Eye trouble: bathe face if afflicted with "tissue growth" in the eyes. Cleansing (magical): use as a spray.Gynecological hemorrhaging: take tea (other ingredients also) following miscarriage (spiritualist prescription).

(Albacar)	Scutellaria sp.	Nueva Leon-Monterrey	Lundell, 1934	
	Ocimum sp.	Zacatecas-Zacatecas	Riley and Trujillo, 1956	Vomiting: boil stems and leaves; take as needed.
19. Albaricoque, Hueso de	Prunus Armeniaca L.	New Mexico-Spanish	Curtin, 1947	Dry nose: grind pit of kernel and place in nostrils (especially for babies). Goiter: apply poultice of ground kernel pit
20. Albayalde	not a plant -- white talc	New Mexico-Spanish	Ford, 1966	
21. Alberjón	Pisum satium [dried peas]	New Mexico-Spanish	Shulman and Smith, 1962	Headache
22. Alberjón de Patito	unidentified [wild peas]	New Mexico-Spanish	Shulman and Smith, 1962	Aire, headaches and dizziness
23. Alcachopa	Cleome sp.	Zacatecas-Zacatecas	Riley and Trujillo, 1956	Liver ailments caused by overdrinking: boil leaves and stems and take infusion twice daily as needed
24. Alcanfor	Cinnamomum camphora Nees and Eberm. [camphor]	New Mexico-Spanish	Curtin, 1947	Rheumatism: rub on joints with whiskey. Headache and faintness: inhale aroma.

Spanish Name	Botanical Name	Location	Reference	Use
		New Mexico-Spanish	Shulman and Smith, 1962	Wounds: treat infections
	Artemisia mexicana	Chihuahua-Tepehuán	Pennington, 1963a	Colds: take tea
25. Alcaparrosa	unidentified white powder ?zinc sulfate	New Mexico-Spanish	Ford, 1966	Asthma (4)
26. Alconfor	unidentified	Durango-El Torreón (near La Ferreria)	Riley and Trujillo, 1956	Ear trouble: apply wet section of herb to ear
27. Alegría	*Amaranthus paniculatus* L.	New Mexico-Spanish	Curtin, 1947	Cosmetic: make facial and apply to protect face from sun. Tuberculosis, heart trouble, jaundice: use to bathe. Heart trouble: boil flowers, strain, sweeten and drink.
	Amaranthus cruentus L.	New Mexico-Spanish	Shulman and Smith, 1962	Retardation: boil with pine, give to help retarded child speak
	Amaranthus cruentus L.	New Mexico-Spanish	Ford, 1966	Heart trouble: grind with cinnamon, Remolino and deer's blood; add to wine and take periodically (3)

28. Alejandria	_Cowania plicata_ D. Don	San Luís Potosí-Charcas	Lundell, 1934	
29. Alfalfa	_Medicago sativa_ L.	New Mexico-Spanish	Curtin, 1947	Bedbug repellent
	Medicago sativa L.	New Mexico-Spanish	Ford, 1966	Stomach pains: use seeds (1)
	Medicago sativa L.	San Luís Potosí-Charcas	Whiting, 1934	For las reses (cattle)
30. Alfalfón	_Melilotus alba_ Desr.	New Mexico-Spanish	Curtin, 1947	Bedbugs: place flowering plant between mattresses. Flies: hang branches in room to attract flies, then remove from house. Linens: use to sweeten them when stored.
31. Alfilerillo	_Erodium cicutarium_ L'Hér.	New Mexico-Spanish	Curtin, 1947	Diuretic: boil and drink. Rheumatism: boil in water and bathe. Gonorrhea: make decoction with Yerba del Burro (_Distichlis spicata_), Piloncillo, drink lukewarm, twice daily.
	Erodium cicutarium L'Hér.	New Mexico-Spanish	Ford, 1966	Urinary disorders: make tea and drink (1)
	Erodium cicutarium L'Hér.	Chihuahua-Juarez	Ford and Ford, 1965	

Spanish Name	Botanical Name	Location	Reference	Use
	Erodium cicutarium L'Hér.	San Luís Potosí-Charcas	Whiting, 1934 Lundell, 1934	Sore throat: boil in water and gargle
	Erodium sp.	Durango-El Torreón near La Ferreria	Riley and Trujillo, 1956	Body sores: grind leaves in fine powder and sprinkle over sore after washing
32. Alfrom-brillo	Verbena elegans var. asperata	Chihuahua-Tepehuán	Pennington, 1963a	Stomach disorders: take as tea. Catarro (influenza): take as tea.
33. Algarroba	Acacia pennatula	Chihuahua-Tepehuán	Pennington, 1963a	Venereal disease: decoct bark and drink
34. Algerita	Berberis trifoliolata	Texas	Kearney and Peebles, 1964	
35. Alhucema	Lavandula spica L. [lavender]	New Mexico-Spanish	Curtin, 1947	Menstrual hemorrhaging: grind and mix with Manzanilla; apply with warm rag. Purification: use as incense in sick room and for mother three days after childbirth. Parturition: fumigate to facilitate difficult birth. Phlegm (in babies): give tea of seeds to nursing mother or chew seeds, place in small bag and put in

				baby's mouth. Colic (in babies, from first milk): apply tea to nipple. Vomiting: take dry leaves. Stomach trouble: take as tea.
	Lavandula sp.	New Mexico-Spanish	Shulman and Smith, 1962	Stomachache: use seed
	Lavandula sp.	New Mexico-Spanish	Ford, 1966	Stomach gas: take as tea (especially for babies) (1). Coughs: take as tea (1).
(Aluzema)	*Lavandula* sp.	New Mexico-Spanish	Van Der Eerden, 1948	Post-partum hemorrhage: smoke patient with dry flower petals or grind into powder, place on cloth and wear as sanitary pad. Tea for babies: give to newborns until colostrum gone from mother.
(Alucema)	*Lavandula* sp.	Nueva Leon-Monterrey	Lundell, 1934	
36. Aliso	*Platanus Wrightii*	Chihuahua-Tarahumar	Pennington, 1963b	Medicinal tea: use bark

Spanish Name	Botanical Name	Location	Reference	Use
37. Almacigo de Sabina	Juniperus monosperma (Engelm.) Sarg.	New Mexico-Spanish	Curtin, 1947	Facial swelling: grind white beans, Mastranso (Marrubium vulgare L.), and this resin and rub on afflicted areas
38. Almorrana	unidentified	Nueva Leon-Monterrey	Lundell, 1934	Medicinal herb
39. Alquitrán	unidentified (resin)	New Mexico-Spanish	Ford, 1966	Incense: burn (3)
(Alquitrán, Flor de)	unidentified	New Mexico-Spanish	Shulman and Smith, 1962	Fever: use as tea
40. Alta Mesa	Chrysanthemum parthenium (L.) Bernh.	Valley of Mexico-Tepotzlan	Redfield, 1928	El daño (local form of evil eye): cook with Tripa de Judas (Parietaria pennsylvanica Muhl.) and give to afflicted children
41. Altamisa	unidentified (aster family)	New Mexico-Spanish	Shulman and Smith, 1962	Stomachache: boil plant without root and use
	Artemisia sp.	New Mexico-Tewa area	Robbins, et al., 1916	Parturition: midwife gives snuff made with Collálle, Punche, and Altamisa
	Tanacetum vulgare L.	New Mexico-Spanish	Ford, 1966	Sometimes confused with and used as Altamisa de la Sierra

	unidentified	Chihuahua-Juarez	Ford and Ford, 1965	
	Parthenium lyratum Gray	San Luís Potosí-Charcas	Whiting, 1934	
	Zaluzania triloba (Ort.) Pres.	San Luís Potosí-Charcas	Whiting, 1934	
42. Altamisa de Castilla	unidentified	Coahuila-Saltillo	Lundell, 1934	Stomachaches
43. Altamisa Mexicana	Chrysanthemum parthenium Pers.	New Mexico-Spanish	Curtin, 1947	Menstrual problems (failure to menstruate): boil in large quantities and use in sitz bath. Also, same uses as listed below for Altamisa de la Sierra.
44. Altamisa de la Sierra	Artemisia franserioides Greene	New Mexico-Spanish	Curtin, 1947	Colic: chew fresh leaves with salt. Colds: grind leaves and make tea. Stomachache: grind leaves and make tea. Diarrhea: grind leaves and make tea. Constipation: make suppositories with this, Punche, Añil del Muerto (Verbesina encelioides), honey, Piloncillo, and laundry soap.

Spanish Name	Botanical Name	Location	Reference	Use
45. Alta Reina (Harta Reina)	*Piqueria trinervia* Cav.	Valley of Mexico-Tepotzlan	Redfield, 1928	Los aires (evil spirits): use with other herbs for washing. Fever: boil with *Malva parviflora*, Yerba de San José (*Verbena polystachya*) and Rosa de Castilla (*Rosa* sp.) and drink infusion.
46. Altea (see also Flor Altea)	*Anoda acerifolia* (Zucc.) DC. *Anoda hastata* Cav.	Western Mexico	Rose, 1899	Stomach inflammation: mix leaves with olive oil and take
47. Alumbre, Piedre	not a plant -- alum	New Mexico-Spanish	Ford, 1966	Burns: apply to affected area (1). Teeth (to tighten): make powder and use in a mouthwash.
48. Aluzema see Alhucema				
49. Alvacar see Albáca				
50. Amapola	*Oenothera triloba* *Oenothera laciniata*	Chihuahua-Tarahumar	Pennington, 1963b	Food: boil leaves, salt, and eat as greens or add to atole

(see also Yerba del Golpe)	<u>Oenothera</u> <u>rosea</u>	Chihuahua-Tepehuán	Pennington, 1963a	Stomach upsets: make tea from whole plant
	<u>Oenothera</u> <u>Greggii</u> var. <u>Pringelei</u> Munz	San Luís Potosí-Charcas	Whiting, 1934	Cough: boil in water
	<u>Galpinsia</u> <u>hartwegi</u> (Benth.) Britton	San Luís Potosí-Charcas	Whiting, 1934	Cough: boil in water
	unidentified	San Luís Potosí-Charcas	Whiting, 1934	Cough: boil in water
	unidentified	Chihuahua-Tepehuán	Pennington, 1963a	Stimulant: make tea from stem and leaves
51. Amargo	unidentified	San Luís Potosí-Charcas	Whiting, 1934	Medicinal plant
52. Amarrio	<u>Prunus</u> <u>armeniaca</u>	San Luís Potosí-Charcas	Whiting, 1934	Food: eat fruit
53. Amole	<u>Yucca</u> sp.	New Mexico-Spanish	Van Der Eerden, 1948	Bathing: use root for soap
	<u>Yucca</u> sp.	New Mexico-Spanish	Ford, 1966	Washing clothes and hair: use roots for soap (1), (3), (5).

Spanish Name	Botanical Name	Location	Reference	Use
	Yucca sp.	New Mexico-Spanish	Curtin, 1947	Washing clothes (especially wool): use root for soap. Stimulant: boil, mash young shoots; cook juice longer; red liquid taken by Penitentes to make them brave. Rheumatism: rub syrup on joints. Gonorrhea: crush root, boil, and take warm tea daily.
	Yucca sp.	New Mexico-Spanish	Shulman and Smith, 1962	Washing: hair and woolens
	Yucca baccata	New Mexico-Tewa area	Robbins et al., 1916	Food: eat fruit. Washing: use root for soap. Fiber: make rope from leaves.
	Agave sp.	Chihuahua, Chihuahua	Zingg, 1932	Washing: use roots for soap
	unidentified	Chihuahua, Juarez	Jones, 1932	Washing hair or clothes: dissolve in hot water
54. Amolillo	*Glycyrrhiza lepidota* Nutt.	New Mexico-Spanish	Curtin, 1947	Post-parturition (to facilitate delivery of the afterbirth): mash roots, froth in water, strain and drink.

				To cleanse uterus: drink liquid unstrained.
55. Amores	<u>Cosmos</u> <u>parviflorus</u> (Jacq.) H.B.K.	New Mexico-Spanish	Curtin, 1947	Purge: take as tea. Chest colds: give tea to children. Whooping cough: take tea of dried flowers.
56. Ámula	"near Ageratum in Eupatoriae"	Coahuila-Torreón	Kelly, 1965	"Bilis": use with other ingredients in a tea for complications related to bilis
57. Anecillo	unidentified	Chihuahua-Parral	Riley and Trujillo, 1956	Body sores: grind leaves in fine powder and sprinkle over sore after washing
58. Angélica	<u>Angelica</u> sp.	Zacatecas-Zacatecas	Riley and Trujillo, 1956	Stomach troubles: boil plant (without root) in water; take as needed
59. Angrelitas	<u>Houstonia</u> <u>acerosa</u> Gray	San Luís Potosí-Charcas	Whiting, 1934	Restrained urine
60. Anís	<u>Pimpinella</u> <u>anisum</u> L.	New Mexico-Spanish	Curtin, 1947	Painful shoulders and chest: toast, grind seeds; mix with whiskey and rub on. Stomach trouble, cough and colic: take seeds as tea. Pneumonia: grind seeds, inmortal and drink with hot water. Carminative: take with Azahar

Spanish Name	Botanical Name	Location	Reference	Use
				and Remolino
	Pimpinella anisum L.	New Mexico-Spanish	Ford, 1966	Colds (to cause sweat to break a cold): take tea made from seeds (3). Heart trouble: see Alegría for recipe (3). Baking: use in sweet rolls and biscochitos (3)
	Pimpinella anisum L.	New Mexico-Spanish	Shulman and Smith, 1962	Aire: see Albacar. Cough or phlegm in children. Colds. Tuberculosis: mix with Brazíl and Copalquín.
	Pimpinella anisum L.	Chihuahua-Juarez	Jones, 1932	Food and beverage: use on bread and in wine making
(Anís Chico)	Pimpinella anisum L.	Nueva Leon-Monterrey	Lundell, 1934	
61. Anís Estrella	Illicium verum	New Mexico-Spanish	Ford, 1966	To calm nerves and aid sleep: take as tea (1). Baking: use as Anís.
62. Anisillo	Tagetes micrantha Cav.	Chihuahua-Chihuahua	Zingg, 1932	Stomach trouble: drink decoction

63. Anisote	Artemisia redolens Artemisia Gray	New Mexico-Spanish	Curtin, 1947	Stomach trouble and colic: chew leaf with salt, wash down with water or boil whole plant to make tea.
64. Añil	Helianthus annuus L.	New Mexico-Tewa area	Robbins et al., 1916	not medicinal
	Helianthus annuus L.	New Mexico-Spanish	Curtin, 1947	Rheumatism: use leaves to prepare bath
65. Añil del Muerto	Verbesina encelioides Cav.	New Mexico-Spanish	Curtin, 1947	Hemorrhoids: powder with punche and apply with warm cloth. Swelling of the lungs and liver trouble: take three times daily ground with sugar, vinegar and cold water.
	Verbesina encelioides (Cav.) Benth.	New Mexico-Spanish	Marquez, 1964	Flatulence: drink tea
	Verbesina encelioides (Cav.) Benth.	New Mexico-Spanish	Ford, 1966	Ulcers: boil whole top of flower in water and drink (3) (1).
	? gold weed aster family	New Mexico-Spanish	Shulman and Smith, 1962	Swelling: boil, take liquid with salt when "one has a swollen body." Laxative.

Spanish Name	Botanical Name	Location	Reference	Use
66. Apio	unidentified	Nueva Leon-Monterrey	Lundell, 1934	Food and medicine: boil
	unidentified	San Luís Potosí-Charcas	Lundell, 1934	Inflammation: use to bathe
67. Aristolochia	<u>Aristolochia</u> sp.	Valley of Mexico-Tepotzlan	Field, 1953	Rheumatism: pulverize, mix with alcohol and ferment. Rub on affected areas before vapor bath. Then rub on again and keep warm.
68. Arnica	<u>Gaillardia nervosa</u> Rydb.	San Luís Potosí-Charcas	Whiting, 1934	Wounds: place flowers in alcohol; apply as needed
	<u>Grindelia oxylepsis</u> Greene	San Luís Potosí-Charcas	Lundell, 1934	
	<u>Heterotheca</u> sp.	Durango-La Ferreria	Riley and Trujillo, 1956	Bruises from blows, falls and swollen legs: boil plant and use as wash or soak
	<u>Aplopoppus spinulosus</u> var. <u>turbinellus</u> (Rydb) Blake		Lundell, 1934	
	unidentified	Durango-Llano Grande (near La Ferreria)	Riley and Trujillo, 1956	Flesh wounds: boil whole plant with root and use as wash

69. Artemisia Yerba	*Artemisia* sp.	New Mexico-Spanish	White, 1941	
70. Artiguilla	*Bouteloua gracilis* (H.B.K.) Lag.	San Luís Potosí-Charcas	Whiting, 1934	
71. Arroz	*Oryza sativa* [rice]	New Mexico-Spanish	Shulman and Smith, 1962	Heart ailments: use to prevent
72. Ascona	unidentified	Zacatecas-Zacatecas	Riley and Trujillo, 1956	Inflammations (internal and external): boil branches and use for bath; make a compress or boil and drink as needed. Sore throat: make infusion and gargle.
73. Atole	*Zea mays* [corn gruel]	New Mexico-Spanish	Shulman and Smith, 1962	Parturition: preferred food after delivery
74. Azafrán	*Carthamus tinctorius* L.	New Mexico-Spanish	Curtin, 1947	Measles: soak flowers in cold water until water is yellow, strain, drink 1/2 glass at a time to bring out rash and reduce fever
	Carthamus tinctorius L.	New Mexico-Spanish	Ford, 1966	Measles: give tea to help them "break out" (3) (1). Fever: take tea (3) (1). Cooking: use as coloring and flavoring in soups, meatballs (3) (1). Dye: use to dye wool yellow (3).

Spanish Name	Botanical Name	Location	Reference	Use
	[false saffron]	New Mexico-Spanish	Shulman and Smith, 1962	Measles: use in tea to make them come out
75. Azahar de Naranjo (Azar)	<u>Citris</u> sp.	New Mexico-Spanish	Ford, 1966	Most ailments: grind flowers, place in warm water and drink (3). Heart trouble: for recipe see Alegría. To calm nerves and aid sleep: make tea and drink (2).
(Flor Asar)	<u>Citris</u> sp.	New Mexico-Spanish	White, 1941	
	<u>Citris</u> sp.	Nueva Leon-Monterrey	Lundell, 1934	
(Asar de Naranjo)		Zacatecas-Zacatecas	Riley and Trujillo, 1956	
see also Flor de Naranjo				
76. Azucarcan (Piedra Azucar)	not a plant -- rock candy	New Mexico-Spanish	Ford, 1966	Food: candy
77. Azucena	<u>Polianthes tuberosa</u> L.	Valley of Mexico-Tepotzlan	Redfield, 1928	Prevention of abortion (which will occur if a pregnant woman gets a sudden craving for a food

				which cannot be satisfied): take potion of this plant, Flor de San Diego (<u>Laelia</u> sp.), sugar and chocolate.
78. Azufre	sulphur	New Mexico-Spanish	Ford, 1966	Most ailments: mix with water and drink (3). Boils: apply powder (3). Suppositories: one of many ingredients (Punche, Manzanilla, Osha, Romerillo, Yerba Bueno, Piloncillo -- grind and mix with honey, tar soap and rolled into shape) (3). Cough: make into syrup with molasses (1).
79. Bachata (see also Yerba del Empacho)	<u>Chorizanthe fimbriata</u> Nutt.	Baja California-Paipai	Owen, 1963	Diarrhea: make tea for infants from small branches
80. Bainora Prieto	<u>Pisonia capitata</u> (S. Wats.) Standley	Chihuahua-Tarahumar	Bennett and Zingg, 1935	Fever: grind leaves with warm water; strain juice into fresh water; warm and drink
81. Baraca (see Flor de Baraca)				

Spanish Name	Botanical Name	Location	Reference	Use
82. Barba de chivo	Clematis Drummondii T. and G.	San Luís Potosí-Charcas	Whiting, 1934	Frightened animals: use leaves. Skin eruptions: press leaf between fingers and rub on affected areas.
	Clematis Drummondii T. and G.	New Mexico	Wooton and Standley, 1915	
83. Barba de coco	Cocos nucifera L.	San Luís Potosí-Charcas	Lundell, 1934	
84. Barba de Maiz	Zea mays	New Mexico-Spanish	Ford, 1966	Urinary disorders: make tea of corn silk and drink as diuretic (1). Witches: they use corn silk to bewitch (3).
85. Barbasco	Croton texensis (Kl.) Muell. Arg.	New Mexico-Spanish	Curtin, 1947	Insecticide: remove bedbugs by placing under mattress or by placing on hot coals to smoke them out in closed room. Earache: place seed in lamb's wool and put in ear. Headache, neuralgia: apply green or dry leaves to head or inhale smoke. Purge: take powder in warm water. Paralysis: use strong infusion to bathe.

	Croton texensis (Kl.) Muell. Arg.	New Mexico-Spanish	Ford, 1966	Rheumatism: grind dry leaves, mix with honey and rub on swollen areas (3)
	Croton sp.	New Mexico-Spanish	Shulman and Smith, 1962	Laxative
86. Barbo	unidentified	New Mexico-Spanish	Shulman and Smith, 1962	Heart trouble: boil with Oja del Aurelia and drink
87. Batamote	_Baccharis glutinosa_ Pers.	Arizona	Kearney and Peebles, 1964	
88. Bavisa (Babisa or Manza)	_Anemopsis californica_ Hook. & Arn.	Chihuahua-Juarez	Jones, 1932	Boils: use infusion as wash
	Anemopsis californica Hook. & Arn.	Chihuahua-Juarez	Ford and Ford, 1965	Sores: use to wash (8)
(Hoja de babisa)	_Anemopsis californica_ Hook.	Chihuahua-Chihuahua	Zingg, 1932	Sores and boils: boil leaves and roots; use decoction as wash
(see also Mata Gusano)	_Cosmos Pringlei_	Chihuahua-Tarahumar	Pennington, 1963b	Headaches: use roots to make tea. Intestinal disorders: make tea from roots. Sores (from maggots or worms): use pulverized roots for poultice.
89. Bejuco de Huico	_Pithecoctenium_ sp.	West Mexico	Rose, 1899	Headache: apply large winged seeds to temples

Spanish Name	Botanical Name	Location	Reference	Use
90. Bellota	_Quercus_ _Emoryi_ Torr.	Southwest United States	Kearney and Peebles, 1964	
91. Bellota de Sabina	_Phoradendron juniperinum_ Engelm.	New Mexico-Spanish	Curtin, 1947	Food: children sometimes eat them
	Juniperus sp.	New Mexico-Spanish	Curtin, 1947	Venereal disease: drink tea from berries. Blood purification: drink tea made from berries. Stomach trouble: drink tea made from berries.
92. Benna dia	_Porophyllum filiforme_ Rydb.	San Luís Potosí-Charcas	Whiting, 1934	Laxative: boil in water and drink
93. Berbena see Verbena				
94. Berbena ocea de Lagayinas	_Guazuma_ _ulmifolia_		Lundell, 1934	
95. Berguensa see Yerba de la Verguensa				
96. Berro	_Radicula_ _nasturtium_ (L.) Britten & Rendle	New Mexico-Spanish	Curtin, 1947	Heart trouble: eat greens. Kidneys: eat greens. Tuberculosis: crush finely in cold water and take.

	Nasturtium officinale	Chihuahua-Tepehuán	Pennington, 1963a	Influenza: take as tea
	Nasturtium officinale	Baja California-Paipai	Owen, 1963	"Therapeutic"
(see also Lantén cimarrón)	Mimulus guttatus	Chihuahua-Tepehuán	Pennington, 1963a	Fever: boil whole plant to make tea
97. Berros	Coreopsis tinctoria Nutt.	Coahuila-Torreon	Kelly, 1965	Food: drink in decoction as substitute for coffee. Lung difficulties: take as emulsion. Kidney complaints: take as tea.
98. Betabeles	Beta sp. [beets]	New Mexico-Spanish	Shulman and Smith, 1962	Kidneys: use to clean
99. Betonia	unidentified	Nueva Leon-Monterrey	Lundell, 1934	Medicinal herb
100. Betónica	Lepechinia spicata	Valley of Mexico-Tepotzlan	Field, 1953	Uterine tumor causing "stoppage": boil 3 hours then drink a glass 3 times a day before meals.
101. Binorama	Acacia farnesiana	Chihuahua-Tarahumar	Bennett and Zingg, 1935	Insect bites: cook bark and spines in water and drink, especially for

Spanish Name	Botanical Name	Location	Reference	Use
				scorpion stings
102. Biznaga	<u>Ferocactus</u> sp.	Chihuahua-Tarahumar	Pennington, 1963b	Food: grind seeds and eat with pinole
	<u>Mammillaria heyderi</u>	Chihuahua-Tarahumar	Bennett and Zingg, 1935	Food: eat fruit. Earache or deafness: remove spines from plant, cut in half, roast in ashes for 4 minutes; then squeeze soft center into ear
103. Bogambilia	<u>Bougainvillea spectabilis</u>	Nueva Leon-Monterrey	Lundell, 1934	Cough: boil with other herbs
104. Boldo	<u>Peumus boldus</u>	Zacatecas-Zacatecas	Riley and Trujillo, 1956	Liver ailments: boil leaves and take twice daily for 3-5 days. Constipation: as above but take 3 times a day for 2-3 days
105. Bolitas Guasima	<u>Guazuma ulmifolia</u>	Nueva Leon-Monterrey	Lundell, 1934	Gonorrhea
106. Bomba (Florefundia)	<u>Datura candida</u>	Valley of Mexico-Tepotzlan	Redfield, 1928	Toothache: coat petals with grease and place on gums
107. Borraja	<u>Borago officinalis</u> L.	New Mexico-Spanish	Ford, 1966	Stomach ailments: take as tea (1). Bites or infections: apply as

				poultice with pork fat (1). Fever: take as tea (2) (1). Eye ailments: strain tea and use as eyewash (1). To aid sleep: take as tea (1).
	<u>Borago</u> <u>officinalis</u> L.	Nueva Leon-Monterrey	Lundell, 1934	Fever
	<u>Borago</u> <u>officinalis</u> L.	San Luís Potosí-Charcas	Lundell, 1934	
	<u>Borago</u> <u>officinalis</u> L.	Valley of Mexico-Tepotzlan	Redfield, 1928	Fever: steep in water and drink.
	<u>Sonchus</u> <u>oleraceus</u> L.	San Luís Potosí-Charcas	Whiting, 1934	
108. Bougainbilla see Flor de Bougainbilla				
109. Brasilillo	<u>Calliandra</u> <u>eriophylla</u>	Chihuahua-Tarahumar	Pennington, 1963b	Gonorrhea: boil plant several hours, strain, set aside for a few days; then drink before eating each morning for 3 months.
110. Brazíl	<u>Haematoxylon</u> <u>Campechianum</u> L.	New Mexico-Spanish	Curtin, 1947	Tuberculosis: drink decoction and use for sponge bath.

Spanish Name	Botanical Name	Location	Reference	Use
				Smallpox: soak chips in cold water until water is red; drink when thirsty to make smallpox break out. Heart trouble: boil in water with Azar, Anís, Alegría strain, add Sangre de Venado, and Coral Preparado; drink before meals.
Palo Brazíl	Caesalpinia sp.	New Mexico-Spanish	White, 1941	
	Caesalpinia echinata	New Mexico-Spanish	Ford, 1966	Heart trouble: add to wine and drink (3)
	? Haematoxylon sp. [logwood]	New Mexico-Spanish	Shulman and Smith, 1962	Heart trouble: boil and drink. Tuberculosis: mix with Anís and Copalquín and use as tonic.
	Haematoxylon brasiletto	Chihuahua-Tarahumar	Pennington, 1963b	Jaundice: crush young branches and decoct into a compound for rubbing on patient. Dye: red.
111. Buena Mujer see Pepapega				
112. Bura dulce	Eysenhardtia polystachya (Orteg.) Sarg.	San Luís Potosí-Charcas	Whiting, 1934	

113. Caballo see Cola de Caballo				
114. Cabellito de Angel	_Ceiba pentandra_ (L.) Gaertn.	Valley of Mexico-Tepotzlan	Redfield, 1928	Coughs: boil flowers with Yerba Dulce (_Lippia dulcis_) and manzanillos (?) and apply externally
115. Ċacachila (Palo Apestoso)	_Karwinskia Humboltiana_	Chihuahua-Tarahumar	Pennington, 1963b	Food: eat berries, as starvation food in June. Fever: crush bark and make tea.
	Karwinskia Humboltiana	Chihuahua-Tepehuán	Pennington, 1963a	Fever: boil bark and take as tea, hot or cold
116. Cachana	unidentified	New Mexico-Spanish	Ford, 1966	Witches: carry or keep pieces of root (unburned) for protection against witches (3). Headache: burn piece of root and inhale (3) (1). Nosebleed: burn piece of root and inhale (1). Tonsilitis: powder root and blow into tonsils to dry them up (1).
	unidentified	Chihuahua-Juarez	Ford and Ford, 1965	Parturition: for mothers after baby is born (8)
(Flor de Cachana)	_Liatris_ sp.	New Mexico-Spanish	Ford, 1966	

Spanish Name	Botanical Name	Location	Reference	Use
(Cochana)	unidentified	New Mexico-Spanish	Shulman and Smith, 1962	Witches: cary odorless root as prophylactic
(Cachano)	_Trixis californica_ Kell.	Coahuila-Torreón	Kelly, 1965	Fertility: take decoction to facilitate conception
117. Cachanilla	_Pluchea sericea_ (Nutt.) Coville	Southwest United States	Goss, 1903	
		Southwest United States	Beal, 1943	Diarrhea and stomachache. Snakebite on horses: use roots.
118. Cadillos	_Xanthium commune_ Britton	New Mexico-Spanish	Curtin, 1947	Diarrhea: boil 3 burrs in a cup of water and drink
				Rattlesnake bite: apply poultice of leaves
(Cadio)	_Xanthium canadense_ Mill.	New Mexico-Spanish	Wooton, 1894	
119. Cal	lime	New Mexico-Spanish	Ford, 1966	Cooking: use to make posole (3). Insecticide: put on plants (3).
120. Calabasa	_Cucurbita muschata_	San Luís Potosí-Charcas	Wooton, 1934	Food: eat fruit
(Calabaza, Semilla de)	_Cucurbita_ sp.	New Mexico-Spanish	Ford, 1966	Food: roast and eat seeds (3)

121. Cala-bazilla	_Cucurbita foetidissima_ H.B.K.	New Mexico-Spanish	Curtin, 1947	Washing hair and clothing: use fruit pulp to help remove grease
	Cucurbita foetidissima H.B.K.	New Mexico-Tewa	Curtin, 1947	Laxative: grind roots, stir in cold water and drink
	Cucurbita foetidissima H.B.K.	New Mexico-Spanish	Curtin, 1947	Rheumatism: a) bake fruit, split and rub afflicted parts; b) mix ground roots with olive oil, aceite de comer and apply. Pains under eyes: grind flowers, powdered Contrayerba (_Kallstroemia_), and Patito del Campo (_Lathyrus_) and rub on affected area. Saddle sores: use decoction of roots. Cathartic: use decoction of roots.
	Cucurbita foetidissima	New Mexico-Spanish	Ford, 1966	Roots are very poisonous (3)
	Cucurbita foetidissima	Arizona	Kearney and Peebles, 1964	Food: fruits eaten
	Cucurbita digitata Gray	Baja California-Paipai	Owen, 1963	"Shamanism"

Spanish Name	Botanical Name	Location	Reference	Use
122. Calaguala	Notholaena candida	Chihuahua-Tarahumar	Bennett and Zingg, 1935	Fever: take decoction
	Notholaena sinuata	Chihuahua-Chihuahua	Zingg, 1932	Inflammation and bruises: drink decoction
also called Negrito	Asplenium monanthes L.	Chihuahua-Tepehuán	Pennington, 1963a	Parturition: steep leaves in hot water, drink when cool, before and immediately after childbirth. Rheumatis pains: take hot tea made from leaves.
123. Calahua del Indio	Notholaena sinuata (Sw.) Kaulf.	Chihuahua-Chihuahua	Zingg, 1932	Inflammation and bruises: drink decoction
124. Calco Meca see Cocolmeca	unidentified	Chihuahua-Juarez	Ford and Ford, 1965	Tea (8)
125. Calampacate	Gnaphalium semiamplexicaule LC.	San Luís Potosí-Charcas	Whiting, 1934	Wounds: apply leaf
126. Camaron see Flor de Camaron				
127. Camote de Monte	Peteria sp.	Texas	Kearney and Peebles, 1964	Food: roots edible

128. Camote de Raton	Hoffmanseggia densiflora Benth.	Arizona	Kearney and Peebles, 1964	Food: roast and eat roots
129. Camotito Blanco	unidentified	Valley of Mexico-Tepotzlan	Field, 1953	Boils (from evil spirits): mix root powder and liquid from boiled flowers with mescal and apply. Toothache: use liquid as rinse.
130. Canaguala see also Cañahuala	Polypodium sp.	Durango-Llano Grande near La Ferreria	Riley and Trujillo, 1956	Internal bruises from blows or injuries: boil plant, add a pinch of sand, allow to set overnight; take before breakfast; repeat making fresh batches and taking them each day for 9 days
	unidentified [fern]	Nueva Leon-Monterrey	Lundell, 1934	Medicinal herb
131. Cancerina	Asclepias sp.	Zacatecas-Zacatecas	Riley and Trujillo, 1956	Sores (infected, genital area in females): boil piece of root and use to bathe, for wet compresses and drink daily before evening meal
132. Candelilla	Euphorbia antisyphilitica Zucc.	Coahuila-Torreón	Kelly, 1965	Vaginal discharge: drink decoction. Venereal disease complaint in men: boil with other plants and drink

Spanish Name	Botanical Name	Location	Reference	Use
	Euphorbia sp.	Zacatecas-Zacatecas	Riley and Trujillo, 1956	Venereal disease: boil stalks and leaves, let set overnight and take before breakfast for 9 days
	unidentified	San Luís Potosí-Charcas	Lundell, 1934	Bladder trouble
133. Canela en Raja	*Cinnamomum zeylanicum*	New Mexico-Spanish	Van der Eerden, 1948	Parturition:(to hasten delivery) give mother 3 sticks or the equivalent in powdered form. Repeat if necessary.
	Cinnamomum sp.	New Mexico-Spanish	Ford, 1966	Colds: take tea to cause sweating (1). Stomachache: add ground cinnamon and sugar to coffee or water and drink (3). Heart trouble: for recipe see Alegría. Canning: use for flavoring, e.g. pears (3)
(Canela)	*Cinnamomum* sp.	New Mexico-Spanish	Shulman and Smith, 1962	Aire: see Albacar. Stomach-ache: mix with warm water and drink. Hemorrhage after delivery : use in tea. Child "feels sick": give in coffee. Susto: use with bicarbonate of soda, spear-mint and nuts.

134. Caña	Saccharum officinarum	Coahuila-Torreón	Kelly, 1965	Food: chew as a sweet
135. Caña de Castilla	Arundo donax	Valley of Mexico-Tepotzlan	Madsen, 1965	Cough caused by cold: make tea with Itamo Real (Pellaea cordata) and leaves of Tejocote (Crataegus mexicana)
136. Cañafístola	Cassia Fistula L.	Coahuila-Torreón	Kelly, 1965	Abortion and/or regulation of menstruation: take decoction with this and other items
(Caña Fistula) see also Caña Pistola	Cassia sp.	Chihuahua-Parral (from Oaxaca?)	Riley and Trujillo, 1956	To clear urine: boil seed pod and seeds in water and take infusion 3 times a day for 9-10 days. Coughs: as above.
137. Cañahuala	Notholaena sinuata var. integerrima Hook.	Chihuahua-Juarez	Jones, 1932	Stomach medicine: make an infusion
138. Cañaigre	Rumex sp.	New Mexico-Cochiti	Lange, 1959	Food: eat young leaves as greens and young stems as rhubarb. Tanning: use roots.
	Rumex hymenosepalus	New Mexico-Spanish	White, 1941	

Spanish Name	Botanical Name	Location	Reference	Use
(Caña Agria)	Rumex hymenosepalus Torr.	New Mexico-Spanish	Curtin, 1947	Tanning: use roots in water to soak skins. Pyorrhea: make rinse of ground root. Sore throat: make gargle from root. Skin irritations: powder root and apply. Skin inflammations: mix roots with Castilleja and alum and apply.
	Rumex hymenosepalus Torr.	New Mexico-Spanish	Ford, 1966	To tighten teeth: use roots for mouthwash (1)
	Rumex sp. ? unidentified	New Mexico-Spanish	Shulman and Smith, 1962	Teeth: chew, good for teeth, to treat pyorrhea
	Rumex hymenosepalus Torr.	Chihuahua-Juarez	Jones, 1932	Stomach medicine and blood tonic
	Rumex hymenosepalus Torr.	Chihuahua-Juarez	Ford and Ford, 1965	Teeth: to clean (8)
139. Caña Pistola see also Cañafistula	Cassia sp.	Zacatecas-Zacatecas	Riley and Trujillo, 1956	Sores and genital inflammations of women: boil pod and use liquid as douche. Whooping Cough: boil pod in water, mix with milk, add sugar, take 2 times a day.

140.	Cañatilla (Cañutillo del Campo)	_Ephedra torreyana_ S. Wats.	New Mexico-Spanish	Curtin, 1947	Venereal disease: take as tea. Fever and Kidney pain (diuretic): take decoction.
	Cañutillo	_Ephedra_ sp.	New Mexico-Spanish	White, 1941	
		Ephedra sp.	New Mexico-Spanish	Ford, 1966	Stomach disorders: take as tea (3). Urinary disorders: take as tea (1).
	Cañatillo, Popotillo	_Ephedra_ sp.	New Mexico	Kearney and Peebles, 1964	Venereal disease and kidney ailments: take tea made from branches
	Cañutillo	_Ephedra_ sp.	Chihuahua-Juarez	Ford and Ford, 1965	Stomach disorders: take as tea (8)
		Ephedra californica Wats.	Baja California-Paipai	Owen, 1963	Venereal disease: take tea
		Equisetum arvense	New Mexico-Tewa area	Robbins, et al., 1916	
	Cañutillo del Llano	_Equisetum hiemale_ L.	New Mexico-Spanish	Curtin, 1947	Gonorrhea
141.	Capitanejo	unidentified	San Luís Potosí-Charcas	Lundell, 1934	Wounds and boils on animals: use as wash
142.	Capulín	_Prunus melanorydbl_ Rydb.	New Mexico-Cochiti	Lange, 1959	Food: eat cherries; make jelly, jam, or meal cakes

Spanish Name	Botanical Name	Location	Reference	Use
	Prunus melanocarpa (A. Nels.) Rydb.	New Mexico-Spanish	Curtin, 1947	Stomach inflammation: make tea from roots, add Piloncillo; take in morning and before each meal. Rheumatism: make red tea from roots to drink and to bathe in. Dyes: green from inner bark (in spring); purple-red from berries. Food: eat fruit in jam, jelly, or make wine.
	Cydonia oblonga Pyrus Cydonia	Chihuahua-Tarahumar	Bennett and Zingg, 1935	Food: eat fruit
also called Granjén	Celtis pallida Torr.	Coahuila-Torreón	Kelly, 1965	Food: eat fruit raw
143. Capulín Pequeña	Prunus capuli	Chihuahua-Tepehuán	Pennington, 1963a	Scratches, stings, inflammations: crush leaves and apply
Capulín, Corteza de	Prunus capuli	Chihuahua-Chihuahua	Zingg, 1932	Colds: boil bark and drink decoction as tea

144. Capulín Silvestre (Flor de Sauz)	Sambucus mexicana Presl	New Mexico-Spanish	Curtin, 1947	Food: make wine. Fever: add dry flowers to water and drink. Paralysis: steep flowers in hot water and add to bath.
145. Carcoma	Milla biflora Cav.	San Luís Potosí-Charcas	Whiting, 1934	Food: eat bulb
146. Cardo	Argemone ochroleuca ssp. ochroleuca	Chihuahua-Tepehuan	Pennington, 1963a	Fleas: use milky excresence from stalk as lotion to kill fleas. Purgative: crush seeds and add to warm water.
147. Cardo Santo	Centaurea Rothrockii Greenman	New Mexico-Spanish	Van der Eerden, 1948	Parturition: chew petals if thirsty during labor and childbirth
	Cirsium undulatum Nutt.	New Mexico-Spanish	Curtin, 1947	Parturition (to hasten delivery): boil roots and give tea. Earache: put juice from mashed roots on cotton and place in ear. Toothache: boil roots and hold hot tea in mouth. Diarrhea: take decoction of roots. Gonorrhea: make decoction from flowers. Broken bones: make poultice of leaves and roots. Stiff neck: apply pulp from mashed leaves.

Spanish Name	Botanical Name	Location	Reference	Use
	Argemone hispida Gray	New Mexico-Spanish	Curtin, 1947	Rheumatism, dropsy, swelling: apply dried roots or prepare bath from whole plant
	A. platyceras Link and Otto	San Luís Potosí-Charcas	Whiting, 1934	
	Cirsium undulatum (Nutt.) Spreng.	Chihuahua-Chihuahua	Zingg, 1932	Swellings: use decoction to bathe
	C. undulatum Gray	San Luís Potosí-Charcas	Lundell, 1934	
	Centaurea americana	Nueva Leon-Monterrey	Lundell, 1934	
148. Caricillo	unidentified	Chihuahua-Tepehuán	Pennington, 1963a	Parturition: make tea of stems to take at childbirth
149. Carricillo	Iresine calea	Valley of Mexico-Tepotzlan	Field, 1953	Fever and to refresh insides: boil with water, lemon, alcohol, sugar candy and drink before meals. Enema: boil plant alone.
150. Carriuela	Ipomea Mexicana	New Mexico-Spanish	Wooton, 1894	

151. Carrizo	*Phragmites* sp.	New Mexico - Tewa area	Robbins, et al. 1916	
	Phragmites sp.	Arizona	Kearney and Peebles, 1964	Food: eat root stalks and seeds
152. Cáscara	*Juliana adstringens*	Valley of Mexico-Tepotzlan	Field, 1953	Liver diseases and la bilis: boil bark in water until half has evaporated; take before meals.
153. Cáscara de Capulín	*Prunus* sp.	New Mexico-Spanish	Ford, 1966	
154. Cáscara de Encino	*Quercus* sp.	New Mexico-Spanish	Ford, 1966	Sores in mouth: apply (1) (see also Encino)
	Quercus sp.	Durango-Varal (near La Ferreria)	Riley and Trujillo 1956	Inflammations of the teeth: boil inner bark, cook and use as mouthwash.
155. Cáscara de Granada	*Punica granatum* L.	Baja California-Paipai	Owen, 1963	Sore throat: take as tea. (No Spanish name given in Owen).
156. Cáscara de Nogal	*Juglans* sp.	New Mexico-Spanish	White, 1941	
	Juglans sp.	New Mexico-Spanish	Ford, 1966	Mouthwash: use bark to prepare (1)

Spanish Name	Botanical Name	Location	Reference	Use
	Juglans sp.	New Mexico-Spanish	Curtin, 1947	Rheumatism: for leg pains, use decoction to bathe
157. Cáscara Sagrada	Rhamnus californica Esch.	Baja California-Paipai	Owen, 1963	Stomachache and vomiting: make tea from leaves. Constipation: boil piece of bark, leave outside overnight, drink in the morning.
	Rhamnus californica Esch.	New Mexico-Spanish	Ford, 1966	Laxative: boil in water and drink (1)
158. Castilla (see Flor de Castilla and Rosa de Castilla)				
159. Cebada (Savada)	Hordeum vulgare L.	San Luís Potosí-Charcas	Whiting, 1934	
160. Cebadilla	Frasera speciosa	New Mexico-Spanish	Curtin, 1947	Fever: mix ground root with hot water, rub on body, wrap in blankets to cause sweating. Purge: take powdered root in warm water or stir stem in glass of milk. Paralysis: grind roasted root

				and rub on affected areas. Headache: grind root with Inmortal and rub on forehead. Cold: snuff up nose at night. Insecticide: (esp. vs. lice) mix powder with lard and apply to head for 12 hours, wash.
	<u>Swertia</u> <u>radiata</u>?	New Mexico-Spanish	Shulman and Smith, 1962	Constipation: use as laxative
161. Cebolla	<u>Allium</u> <u>cepa</u> L.	New Mexico-Spanish	Curtin, 1947	Chilblains: roast and apply hot in small sections. Teething: babies chew stems and leaves to reduce pain and swelling.
		New Mexico-Spanish	Shulman and Smith, 1962	Wounds: apply. Colds: use to prevent.Pneumonia: to treat and to prevent. TB: in a solution of water and vinegar. Influenza: treat with in a solution of water and vinegar. Fever and chest congestion: stew.
162. Cebollita del Campo	<u>Allium</u> <u>recurvatum</u> Rydb.	New Mexico-Spanish	Curtin, 1947	Flatulence:chew. Fever: mash, soak in water, strain, and drink liquid. Food: eat raw or cooked.
(Sevollita del Campo)	<u>A.</u> <u>Kunthii</u> G. Don. <u>A.</u> <u>scaposum</u> Benth.	San Luís Potosí-Charcas	Whiting, 1934	

Spanish Name	Botanical Name	Location	Reference	Use
163. Cedro	*Juniperus scopulorum* Sarg.	New Mexico-Tewa area	Robbins et al., 1916	
	Cupressus benthamii Endl.	San Luís Potosí-Charcas	Whiting, 1934	"Cultivated."
164. Cedro Colorado	*Juniperus* sp.	New Mexico	Tidestrom and Kittell 1941	
165. Cedrón	*Aloysia triphylla*	Valley of Mexico-Tepotzlan	Madsen, 1965	Anger sickness: for recipe see Ajenjo. Stomachache from eating custard apples: take as tea.
	Lippia triphylla (L 'Hér.) Kuntze	San Luís Potosí-Charcas	Whiting, 1934	Colic in women: boil in water
(Cedrón de Castilla)	*Lippia triphylla* (L 'Hér.) Kuntze	San Luís Potosí-Charcas	Lundell, 1934	Colic: boil in water
	Lippia triphylla (L 'Hér.) Kuntze	Coahuila-Monterrey	Lundell, 1934	Colic
	Lippia triphylla (L 'Hér.) Kuntze	Nueva Leon-Monterrey	Lundell, 1934	Colic
	Lippia sp.	Zacatecas-Zacatecas	Riley and Trujillo, 1956	Chest pains: boil leaves and branches and take liquid twice daily

166. Celantillo	Adiantum capillus-veneris L.	Western Mexico	Rose, 1899	Colic: take as tea. Amenorrhea: take as tea.
167. Cenizo	unidentified	New Mexico-Spanish	Ford, 1966	
	Atriplex canescens (Pursh) Nutt.	Arizona	Kearney and Peebles, 1964	
	unidentified	Chihuahua-Juarez	Ford and Ford, 1965	
	Leucophyllum zygophyllum Johnst.	Coahuila-Torreón	Kelly, 1965	Stomachache: take in tea with other items. Diabetes: take decoction. Bilis: use for tea and herb bath.
(Seniso)	Leucophyllum laevigatum Standl.	San Luís Potosí-Charcas	Lundell, 1934	Medicinal herb
168. Cidra	Citris medica	Chihuahua-Tarahumar	Bennett and Zingg, 1935	Food: fruit not edible raw
169. Cilantro (Culantro)	Coriandrum sativum L.	New Mexico-Spanish	Curtin, 1947	Food: use as seasoning. Pyorrhea and toothache: boil in water and hold in mouth. Cold in stomach: boil and drink. Headache: burn seeds and inhale fumes
		New Mexico-Spanish	Shulman and Smith, 1962	Aire: see Albacar.

Spanish Name	Botanical Name	Location	Reference	Use
	Coriandrum sativum L.	New Mexico-Spanish	Ford, 1966	Sedative: take as tea (1). Food: use to season soup (fresh leaves); use seeds in tamales and carne adovado (3).
	Coriandrum sativum L.	Baja California-Paipai	Owen, 1963	Menstrual difficulties: steep seeds in hot water, drink tea, may also add Rosa de Castilla
171. Cimonillo	Unidentified	San Luís Potosí-Charcas	Whiting, 1934	To give appetite
172. Cinco Llagas	_Zinnia grandiflora_ Nutt.	Chihuahua-Chihuahua	Zingg, 1932	Diarrhea: drink decoction as an astringent
173. Cinco de Mayo	_Amaranthus leucocarpus_ Wats.	New Mexico	Tidestrom and Kittell, 1941	
174. Cinco Yagay	_Tagetes_ sp.	San Luís Potosí-Curtin	Lundell, 1934	
175. Ciruelo del Campo	_Thryallis glauca_	Chihuahua-Tarahumar	Pennington, 1963b	Food: eat fruits. Diarrhea: make tea from leaves. Wounds: use tea as wash.
176. Clamaclancle (see Flor de Clamaclancle				

177.	Clameria	<u>Potentilla</u> <u>Thurberi</u>	Chihuahua-Tepehuán	Pennington, 1963a	Aching gums: crush interior of roots and place between cheek and gums
	(Cloradia, Ratania, Sarasapa-rilla	<u>Krameria</u> sp.	Zacatecas-Zacatecas	Riley and Trujillo, 1956	Kidney ailments and diseases of urinary tract: boil roots and take liquid before breakfast for 9 days. To strengthen blood: make a wine using boiled roots, sugar and alcohol, take after meals for 15 days.
178.	Clavel Blanca	[white carnation]	Durango-Llano Grande	Riley and Trujillo, 1956	Headaches: boil wood ticks in oil until oil turns red, shred a flower and mix, apply to temples. Nosebleed: apply above to mid-face area.
179.	Clavelina	<u>Saponaria</u> <u>offici-nalis</u> L.	New Mexico-Spanish	Curtin, 1947	Washing: use roots as soap
180.	Clavo	<u>Caryophyllus</u> <u>armomaticus</u>	New Mexico-Spanish	Shulman and Smith, 1962	Earache: put in ear with olive oil. Cough: use in hot water.
	(Clavo Entero)	<u>Caryophyllus</u> <u>armomaticus</u>	New Mexico-Spanish	Ford, 1966	Food: use as spice in cook-ing and baking. Toothache: wrap with fat and place in cavity (1) (7).
182.	Cocolméca (Raiz de China)	<u>Salix</u> <u>mexicana</u>	Zacatecas-Zacatecas	Riley and Trujillo, 1956	Blood tonic: take infusion of root 3 times/day for 9

Spanish Name	Botanical Name	Location	Reference	Use
				days. Inflammations of genitals (internal, in women): use infusion of root as douche daily for 9 days.
183. Codo de Fraile	_Thevetia thevatioides_	Zacatecas-Zacatecas	Riley and Trujillo, 1956	Rectal sores: crush interior of the pit of the fruit, mix with lard and apply
184. Cola de Caballo	_Equisetum laevigatum_	Chihuahua-Tarahumar	Pennington, 1963b	Chest ailments: use stems to make tea
	Equisetum laevigatum	Chihuahua-Tepehuán	Pennington, 1963a	Stomach cramps: use stems to make tea
(Caballo)	_Equisetum_ sp.	Chihuahua-Juarez	Ford and Ford, 1965	Kidneys: good for kidneys (8)
	E. hiemale L.	Chihuahua-Chihuahua	Zingg, 1932	Kidney pains: drink decoction
(Carisillo, Cañolilla)	_Equisetum_ sp.	Zacatecas-Zacatecas	Riley and Trujillo, 1956	Kidney, urinary, and venereal diseases: boil and take twice daily for 9 days
185. Cola de Gato	_Heliocereus speciosus_ Britton and Rose	Valley of Mexico-Tepotzlan	Redfield, 1928 Field, 1953	Colds: boil flowers and drink infusion
186. Cola de Ratón	_Muhlenbergia Emersleyi_	Chihuahua-Tarahumar	Pennington, 1963b	

187.	Colita de Rata (Colita de Ratón)	*Eriogonum racemosum* Nutt.	New Mexico-Spanish	Curtin, 1947	Tooth cleaning: use stems
	Colita de Ratón	*Eriogonum* sp.?	New Mexico-Spanish	Shulman and Smith, 1962	Unspecified "remedy"
188.	Collálle (Escoba de la Vibora), (Yerba de la Vibora)	*Gutierrezia sarothrae* (Pursh) Britt. and Rusby	New Mexico-Spanish	Van der Eerden, 1948	Post-partum involution of the uterus: take as tea to help reduce womb to normal size
	(see also Escoba de la Vibora)	*Gutierrezia tenuis* Greene	New Mexico-Spanish	Curtin, 1947	Colic: make poultice with Yerba del Lobo (*Helenium*). Rheumatism: use tea to drink and for bath. Piles: use tea to bathe sore areas. Stomach ache: boil greens or flowers and take as tea. Malaria: decoct greens and use to bathe. Womb trouble and as menostatic: take in a mixture.
		G. linoides *G. longifolia*	New Mexico-Tewa area	Robbins et al., 1916	Parturition and painful menstruation: use to fumigate
		G. sarothrae	New Mexico-Spanish	Ford, 1966	Rheumatism: mix with Yerba del Caballo (*Senecio*?) and water for a bath (3)

Spanish Name	Botanical Name	Location	Reference	Use
	G. sarothrae	New Mexico-Spanish	Marquez, 1964	Menstrual cramping and diarrhea (esp. after childbirth): use to make tea with Yerba Buena and Estafiate
189. Collate	Unidentified	Chihuahua-Juarez	Ford and Ford, 1965	Stomachache: take as tea (8)
190. Colorin (Chilicote), (Chilocote)	_Erythrina flabelliformis_	Chihuahua-Tarahumar	Pennington, 1963b	See Chilocöte
	Erythrina flabelliformis	Chihuahua-Tepehuán	Pennington, 1963a	See Chilocote
191. Colpaquin	?_Picramnia_ sp. or ? _Cinchona_ sp. (see also Copalquin)	Zacatecas-Zacatecas	Riley and Trujillo, 1956	Fever (esp. malaria): soak pieces of bark until soft, make into tablets and take 2 times/day or boil tablet and drink liquid. Sores: mix powdered bark with water and use to wash.
192. Comino	_Cuminum cyminum_ L.	New Mexico-Spanish	Shulman and Smith, 1962	Sore throat: use with ground Contrayerba (caltrop) nuts, and sugar. Aire: mix with Contrayerba cinnamon and nuts, rub on afflicted places.

		New Mexico-Spanish	Ford, 1966	Food: use as cooking spice, add to red chile (3)
	C. cyminium	Chihuahua-Juarez	Jones, 1932	Food: use in sausage
193. Concha (see also Marrubio, Mastranzo)	*Marrubium vulgare* L.	Baja California-Paipai	Owen, 1963	Coughs and colds: take as tea
194. Consuelda	*Taraxacum* sp. *T. taraxacum* (W&S)	New Mexico-Tewa area	Robbins et al., 1916	Food: eat young leaves as greens. Broken bones: make paste of leaves to dress fracture. Bruises: apply ground leaves with dough.
195. Contrayerba	*Kallstroemia* sp.	New Mexico-Spanish	White, 1941	
	Kallstroemia brachystylis Vail	New Mexico-Spanish	Curtin, 1947	Swollen gums: soak powdered root in warm water and use for wash. Sore eyes: same as above. Fever: take tea made from root. Dysentery: same as above. Stomach trouble: same as above. Diarrhea: use with Oshá and Peruvian red bark for tea. Facial pains under eyes: see Calabazilla.
	Kallstroemia sp.? (caltrop family)	New Mexico-Spanish	Shulman and Smith, 1962	Sore throat: grind roots, add sugar and nuts, eat. Aire: mix with comino seed, cinnamon and nuts, rub on

Spanish Name	Botanical Name	Location	Reference	Use
				afflicted place. Rash: good for rash, of smallpox and chickenpox.
	Kallstroemia Californica (Wats.) Vail var. _brachystylis_ Vail	New Mexico-Spanish	Ford, 1966	Tic: grind, sift, and rub on affected area (3)
	Kallstroemia californica (Wats.) Vail var. _brachystylis_ Vail	New Mexico-Santa Clara	Robbins, et al., 1916	Diarrhea: use roots in remedy
	Psoralea pentaphylla	Chihuahua-Tepehuán	Pennington, 1963a	Fever: use leaves for tea
	Psoralea sp.	Chihuahua-Tepehuán	Pennington, 1963a	Fever: use leaves for tea
	Poinsettia radicans	Chihuahua-Tepehuán	Pennington, 1963a	Fever: use tea from plant
	Psoralea pentaphylla L.	San Luís Potosí-Charcas	Whiting, 1934	Stomach trouble: peel and eat root
	Psoralea pentaphylla L.	Valley of Mexico-Tepotzlan	Field, 1953	Typhoid fever, malaria, penumonia: powder root, add alcohol, drink before meals. Labor pains: apply locally to back. To

				facilitate delivery of baby and after birth: rub hard on back and stomach. Diarrhea: add powder to milk, give to children.
	Kallstroemia sp. (caltrop family)	New Mexico-Spanish		Sore throat: grind roots, add sugar and nuts, eat. Aire: mix with comino seed, cinnamon and nuts, rub on afflicted place. Rash: good for rash, smallpox, chickenpox.
196. Contra Yerba de la Sierra	Asclepias sp. af. quinquedentata	Chihuahua-Tepehuán	Pennington, 1963a	Fever
197. Copalquín	Cinchona sp.? [Peruvian red bark]	New Mexico-Spanish	Shulman and Smith, 1962	Tuberculosis: mix with Anís and Brazíl and use as tonic
	Hintonia latiflora Coutarea latiflora	Chihuahua-Tarahumar	Pennington, 1963b	Fever: use bark to make tea
	Hintonia latiflora Coutarea latiflora	Chihuahua-Tarahumar	Pennington, 1963b	Acidity: take decoction

Spanish Name	Botanical Name	Location	Reference	Use
	Hintonia latiflora *Coutarea pterosperma*	Chihuahua-Tarahumar	Bennett and Zingg, 1935	Fever: take decoction. Gall sores (of animals): apply powdered leaves.
	Hintonia latiflora *Coutarea pterosperma*	Chihuahua-Tepehuán	Pennington, 1963a	Fever: take tea made from bark. Influenza: same as above. Sores and snakebites: use tea as cleansing lotion.
	Hintonia sp.?	Chihuahua-Juarez	Ford and Ford, 1965	Stomach: good for stomach (8)
198. Copalquín, Corteza de	unidentified	Chihuahua-Parral	Riley and Trujillo, 1956	Chest pains from blow or injury or stomach pains caused internally: boil and take as needed
199. Coral Preparado	not a plant ? ground sea coral or similar orange colored chalky compound	New Mexico-Spanish	Ford, 1966	Heart trouble: mix with deer's blood, gold leaf, and wine (1a)
200. Corales	not a plant red-orange sea coral beads	New Mexico-Spanish	Ford, 1966	Evil eye: place bracelets of coral on babies to protect against evil eye (3)
201. Coralillo	*Arctostaphylos uva-ursi* (L.)	New Mexico-Spanish	Curtin, 1947	Venereal disease: boil plant, add Piloncillo

	Spreng.			drink each morning for 10 days. Rheumatism: use decoction to bathe. Anemia: boil plant (except root) and take tea before breakfast. Stomach trouble: take tea.
	Anagallis arvensis L.	Valley of Mexico-Tepotzlan	Redfield, 1928	Inflammations: boil leaves and apply
202. Corcomeca	*Phaseolus Metcalfei*	Chihuahua-Tarahumar	Pennington, 1963b	Stomach upset: use roots for tea. Food: use as tesguino catalyst.
203. Cordoncillo	*Elytraria imbricata*	Chihuahua-Tarahumar	Pennington, 1963b	Fever: make tea of leaves. Diarrhea: make tea of leaves. Wounds: make wash from whole plant for washing.
204. Coronilla	*Gaillardia pinnatifida* Torr.	New Mexico-Spanish	Curtin, 1947	Infertility; boil plant (except flower), add Piloncillo strain and drink before meals. Cold and headache: mash stems with salt and water; apply to forehead or temples or make powder from flowers and apply. Anemia: take as tea. Rheumatism: use roots with those of Zarza (*Humulus*) and Yerba de

Spanish Names	Botanical Names	Location	Reference	Use
				Caballo (*Senecio*) for bathing solution
	Berlandiera lyrata var. *macrophylla*	Chihuahua-Tarahumar	Pennington, 1963b	Purgative: make tea from roots
	Tagetes lucida	Chihuahua-Tarahumar	Bennett and Zingg, 1935	Pneumonia
	Berlandiera sp.	Chihuahua-Tepehuan	Pennington, 1963a	Stomach disorders: crush roots, boil in water, and take as tea
205. Corpus	*Magnolia* sp.	Western Mexico	Rose, 1899	Bites (scorpion): use flowers to make tea
206. Costomate	*Physalis? pubescens*	San Luís Potosí-Charcas	Lundell, 1934	
207. Cota	*Thelesperma gracile* A. Gray *Thelesperma longipes* A. Gray *T. longipes* A. Gray	New Mexico-Spanish	Curtin, 1947	Food: boil plant for tea. Dye: boil plant. Diuretic: take as tea. Vermifuge: take as tea. Fever: take as tea-strong with sugar. Chafed skin (babies): give tea and use to bathe.
	T. trifidum	New Mexico-Tewa area	Robbins, et al., 1916	Food: drink tea

	Thelesperma sp.? wild tea [aster family]	New Mexico-Spanish	Shulman and Smith, 1962	Tonic. Beverage. Kidneys: good for kidneys. Bedwetting: use to cure.
208. Crisanta	*Chrysanthemum indicum* L.	New Mexico-Spanish	Curtin, 1947	Stomachache: chew leaf or make tea from leaves
209. Crisantemo	*Chrysanthemum indicum* L.	New Mexico-Spanish	Curtin, 1947	See Crisanta
210. Crucillo	*Randia* sp. or ?*Candalia* sp.	Zacatecas-Zacatecas	Riley and Trujillo, 1956	Indigestion: boil part of fruit in water and take liquid each morning for 9 days
211. Cuasia	*Quassia amara* L.?	New Mexico-Spanish	White, 1941	
Cuacia, Corteza de	unidentified	Chihuahua-Parral (from Oaxaca?)	Riley and Trujillo, 1956	Stomach upsets: soak bark in water and take 3x daily
	unidentified	Chihuahua-Juarez	Jones, 1932	Stomach upset from anger: soak in water and drink liquid
	Picrasma excelsa ?	Nueva Leon-San Luís Potosí	Lundell, 1934	
	Quassia amara L.	Mexico	Martinez, 1959	Stomach ailments. Intestinal parasites.
212. Cuaute-comate	*Crescentia alata*	Valley of Mexico-Tepepan	Madsen, 1965	Pneumonia: take tea made from this and other "hot"

Spanish Name	Botanical Name	Location	Reference	Use
				plants e.g., Itamo and Tejocote
213. Cuipa de Sabina	Juniperus sp.	New Mexico-Spanish	Curtin, 1947	Skin rash (from high blood pressure): boil bark in water, cool, strain, add soda and salt, use for sponge bath
214. Culantrillo	Adiantum capil-lus-veneris L. S-V	Nueva Leon-Monterey	Lundell, 1934	Boil
	Adiantum capil-lus-veneris L. S-V	San Luís Potosí-Charcas	Lundell, 1934	Retarded menstruation: boil in water and take with another item (un-identified)
215. Culantro see Cilantro				
216. Chacate	Krameria sp.	Arizona-Papago	Kearney and Peebles, 1964	Sore eyes: use infusion of twigs. Dye: use roots
	Krameria grayi Rose and Painter K. Canescens Gray	New Mexico	Havard, 1885	Dye: use infusion of bark of root to dye leather brownish-red
217. Chamiso	Atriplex canescens Pursh	New Mexico-Spanish	Curtin, 1947	Stomach pains: chew leaves with salt, take swallow of water
218. Chamiso amarillo	Chrysothamnus sp.? (rabbit brush)	New Mexico-Spanish	Shulman and Smith, 1962	Rheumatic pains: use to bathe afflicted area

219. Chamiso Blanco	Atriplex canescens	Baja California-Paipai	Owen, 1963	Skin eruptions: for recipe see Yerba Santa. Deep pains in bones or muscles: burn fruit and place on sore places.
	Chrysothamnus graveolens, Nutt.	New Mexico-Spanish	Curtin, 1947	Fever: take as tea. Dye: use flowers to make yellow dye.
	Chrysothamnus sp.? [rabbit brush]	New Mexico-Spanish	Shulman and Smith, 1962	Rheumatic pains: use to bathe afflicted parts
220. Chamiso Cimarron	Chrysothamnus graveolens (Nutt.) Greene	New Mexico-Spanish	Curtin, 1947	Fever: take as tea. Dye: use flowers to make yellow dye.
221. Chamiso Colorado	Adenostema sparsi-folium	Baja California-Paipai	Owen, 1963	Toothache: use tea of green leaves for mouth-wash
222. Chamiso Hediondo	Artemisia tri-dentata Nutt. A. Bigelovii Gray	New Mexico-Spanish	Curtin, 1947	Colds and high fever: boil plant and use to bathe. Stomach pains: crush fresh leaves, strain, drink in warm water. Hemorrhaging: take tea of leaves and use also to bathe wounds (especially Penitentes). Rheumatism and Croup and

Spanish Name	Botanical Name	Location	Reference	Use
				chest cold pains: drink and bathe in strong tea of leaves. Influenza: take tea with brandy as part of treatment.
(see Estafiate)	*A. tridentata* Nutt.	New Mexico-Tewa area	Robbins, et al., 1916	Indigestion and flatulence:chew and swallow leaves
223. Chamiso Pardo	*Chrysothamnus sp.*? [dark rabbit brush]	New Mexico-Spanish	Shulman and Smith, 1962	Rheumatic pains: use tea
224. Chan (Chía)	*Salvia reflexa* Hornem.	New Mexico-Spanish	Curtin, 1947	Bedbugs: repellent. Eye (foreign particle in): place seed in eye to help remove particle. Stomach trouble: chew leaves or take decoction. Colic: boil in water with a little Cal (lime).
225. Chante Pusi	*Rhynchosia pyramidalis*	Chihuahua-Tarahumar	Pennington, 1963b	Rheumatism or backache: apply poultice of ground seeds and fat
226. Chaparro Prieto	*Acacia constricta* Benth.	Coahuila-Torreón	Kelly, 1965	Ear ailments: use blossom as cotton to place in ear to collect draining pus
227. Charrsasquilla	unidentified	Nueva Leon-Monterrey	Lundell, 1934	Medicinal herb

228. Chayotillo	Selaginella cuspidata Spreng.	Valley of Mexico-Tepotzlan	Redfield, 1928 Field, 1953	"Loosening of the female organs", a disease of pregnancy: take tea to "fix placenta"
229. Chía	Salvia sp.	New Mexico-Spanish	White, 1941	
	Salvia reflexa Hornem.	New Mexico-Spanish	Curtin, 1947	see Chan
	S. columbariae	Arizona-Pima	Kearney and Peebles, 1964	Food: use seeds to make pinole and a drink. Poultices: use seeds
	S. hispanica	Arizona-Pima	Kearney and Peebles, 1964	
230. Chicalote	Argemone sp.	Arizona	Kearney and Peebles, 1964	
231. Chicascle (see Flor de Chicascle)				
232. Chichiquelita	Solanum podiflorum	Chihuahua-Tepehuán	Pennington, 1963a	Vermifuge: use leaves to make strong tea. Sores (from worms) on men or animals: make lotion from leaves.
	S. nigrum	Chihuahua-Tepehuán	Pennington, 1963a	
	Chenopodium sp.	Arizona-Pima	Curtin, 1947	Food: eat as greens

Spanish Name	Botanical Name	Location	Reference	Use
	unidentified	Chihuahua-Tarahumar	Pennington, 1963b	Purgative: use leaves to prepare tea along with 2 other plants
233. Chico	*Lycium pallidum* Miers	New Mexico-Spanish	Curtin, 1947	Food: eat fruit raw or in stews
234. Chicória	*Taraxacum officinale* Web.	New Mexico-Spanish	Curtin, 1947	Heart trouble: boil flowers until water is yellow; let stand outside overnight; take before breakfast each morning for a month. Blood purification: eat greens raw or cooked with vinegar or make wine and drink
235. Chícura	*Franseria* sp.	Chihuahua-Tepehuán	Pennington, 1963a	Parturition: if difficult take tea made from leaves
	F. ambrosioides Cav.	Arizona-Pima	Curtin, 1947	Menstrual pain and hemorrhage: crush and boil roots, strain, cool outside overnight, take at breakfast
236. Chile (chili)	*Capsicum annuum*	New Mexico-Spanish	Shulman and Smith, 1962	Cold or pneumonia: split, boiled, place on back to cause sweating. Stomach: good for stomach. Tuberculosis: eat to prevent. Blood: good for the blood.

	Capsicum annuum C. frutescens L.	San Luís Potosí-Charcas	Whiting, 1934	Food: use in cooking
237. Chile Puerco	Amaranthus blitoides S. Wats.	New Mexico-Spanish	Curtin, 1947	Sunburn: crush plant, add water, and wash skin to bleach. Food: eat young leaves as greens.
238. Chilicote (Colorín)	Erythrina flabelliformis Kearney	Arizona	Kearney and Peebles, 1964	
	Erythrina flabelliformis Kearney	Chihuahua-Tepehuan	Pennington, 1963a	Purgative: use seeds in small amounts
	Erythrina flabelliformis	Chihuahua-Tarahumar	Pennington, 1963b	Intestinal disorders: toast, grind red beans, mix with water, take a little as an emetic. Toothache: use crushed beans.
239. Chilicoyote	Cucurbita foetidissima H.B.K.	New Mexico-Spanish	Curtin, 1947	see Calabazilla
240. Chilille	Polygonum hydropiper	New Mexico	Tidestrom and Kittell, 1941	
(Chilillo)	Polygonum hydropiperoides	Valley of Mexico-Tepepan	Madsen, 1965	Piles: rub sore area with milky fluid from stalk
241. Chillipiquin	Capsicum baccatum L.	Arizona	Kearney and Peebles, 1964	Food: use as condiment. Local stimulant: use berries.

Spanish Name	Botanical Name	Location	Reference	Use
242. Chilti-piquín	*Capsicum annuum* *C. frutescens*	Chihuahua-Tarahumar	Bennett and Zingg, 1935	Food: use to make sauce and relish. Curing ceremony: for fields, animals, and death ceremony
243. Chimaja	*Aulospermum purpureum* S. Wats.	New Mexico-Spanish	Curtin, 1947	Food: eat roots raw; use leaves for seasoning. Debility and stomach trouble: boil dry leaves and flowers and drink tea 3 times a day.
	Cymopterus purpureus S. Wats.	New Mexico-Spanish	Ford, 1966	Stomachache: chew leaves (3). Food: eat roots raw; use leaves to flavor beans and dried peas (3).
	Cymopterus sp.? [Indian parsley]	New Mexico-Spanish	Shulman and Smith, 1962	Stomachache: use. Flatulence: use as flavoring for peas and beans to prevent gas
244. Chiquete de Embarañada (Chicote Embarañada)	*Lygodesmia juncea* Pursh	New Mexico-Spanish	Curtin, 1947	Gum: chew small yellow balls
245. Chocoyle (Jocoyol) (Socoyol)	*Oxalis violacea* L.	New Mexico-Spanish	Curtin, 1947	Food: eat raw. Vermifuge: boil leaves in water and take.

246. Cholla	Opuntia parryi Engelm.	Baja California-Paipai	Owen, 1963	Diarrhea: make tea of root and another item
	Opuntia sp.	Baja California-Kiliwa	Meigs, 1939	Food: eat seeds as pinole
247. Chuchaca	Erigonum tenellum Torr.	Chihuahua-Chihuahua	Zingg, 1932	Purgative: boil and drink decoction
248. Chuchupate	Ligusticum Porteri C. and R.	New Mexico-Spanish	Curtin, 1947	See Osha
(Chuchufate) (see also Osha)	Ligusticum Porteri	Chihuahua-Tarahumar	Pennington, 1963b	Rheumatism: boil crushed roots and use as wash. Stomach disorders: use tea made from crushed roots and leaves.
249. Chuchupostle (Angélica)		Chihuahua-Parral	Riley and Trujillo, 1956	Stomach ailments, rheumatism, body sores, and animal bites: take infusion of root.
250. Chupón	Castilleja sp.	Chihuahua-Tepehuán	Pennington, 1963a	Urination (to stimulate): take as tea
	unidentified	Chihuahua-Tepehuán	Pennington, 1963a	Fever: take as tea
251. Cuscuta	Cuscuta curta Engelmann	New Mexico-Santo Domingo	Curtin, 1947	Bites (insect): boil and drink or burn in old yucca flower stalk to fumigate bites and

Spanish Name	Botanical Name	Location	Reference	Use
				reduce irritation.
252. Damiana	Turnera humifusa (Presl) Endlich	West Mexico	Rose, 1899	Stomach and intestinal pains: take as tea
	Chrysactinia mexicana Gray	Chihuahua-Chihuahua	Zingg, 1932	Pregnancy: boil and drink tea as aid during pregnancy
	Heliotropium Greggii Torr.	Coahuila-Torreón	Kelly, 1965	Infertility:use in decoction with other items to "heat" womb
253. Dátil	Yucca sp.	New Mexico-Spanish	Curtin, 1947	see Amole
	Y. baccata	New Mexico-Spanish	Robbins, et al., 1916	see Amole
254. Diente de Culebra	Serjania mexicana	Chihuahua-Tarahumar	Pennington, 1963b	Bruises, sprains, fractures: crush stems and use for poultice. Fertility: bruise white flowers and stems to make tea; take until conception occurs
255. Diente de Vibora	Serjania mexicana	Chihuahua-Tarahumar	Bennett and Zingg, 1935	Pain and rheumatism: remove prickles, cut stem in half, and place next to skin and/or on affected areas

256. Digerillo	Ricinus communis L.	Valley of Mexico-Tepotzlan	Redfield, 1928	Fever: boil leaves and take tea
257. Dormilón	Rudbeckia laciniata L.	New Mexico-Spanish	Curtin, 1947	Gonorrhea: take strong tea made from leaves each morning. Emmenagogue: same as above, for 9 days.
	Rudbeckia tagetes James	New Mexico-Spanish	Curtin, 1947	Cold congestion: crush wet roots or grind dry ones and take with cold water 3 times a day. Female trouble.
	Verbena macdougalii Heller	New Mexico-Spanish	Curtin, 1947	Diuretic: take as tea. Toothache: mash green leaves and place on gums and cheek.
	Rudbeckia sp.? or Ratibida sp. [cone flower]	New Mexico-Spanish	Shulman and Smith, 1962	unspecified "remedy"
258. Drago	Pterocarpus acapulcensis Rose	Nueva Leon-Monterrey	Lundell, 1934	
259. Durazno	Prunus persica	New Mexico-Spanish	Curtin, 1947	Purge: use flowers. Fever: boil bark and take tea hot or cold. Asthma: take tea made from leaves. Menstrual troubles: use tea as douche.

Spanish Name	Botanical Name	Location	Reference	Use
	Prunus persica	New Mexico-Spanish	Shulman and Smith, 1962	Fever. Infection: "good for combatting infection."
	unidentified	San Luís Potosí-Charcas	Whiting, 1934	Food: eat fruit
(Durazno, Oja de)	Prunus persica?	New Mexico-Spanish	Shulman and Smith, 1962	"Cancer" sores: bathe sores with peach water
260. Egara	Ficus carica L.	San Luís Potosí-Charcas	Whiting, 1934	Food: eat fruit
261. Embarrañada (Yerba de la Tusa)	Lepachys tagetes A. Gray	New Mexico-Spanish	Curtin, 1947	Toothache: apply powdered root. Red pustules boil in water and use to bathe. Rheumatism: same as above
262. Encina	Quercus sp.	New Mexico	Tidestrom and Kittell, 1941	
263. Encinillo	Quercus fendleri Liebm.	New Mexico-Spanish	Curtin, 1947	Blood (to give strenth): make tea of leaves and drink warm. Anemia: drink tea cold.
	unidentified	Durango-Llano Grande near La Ferreria	Riley and Trujillo, 1956	Hair dandruff and lice: boil leaves in water and use as rinse after shampoo

(Encinilla)	Croton monanthogynus Michx.	Chihuahua-Chihuahua	Zingg, 1932	Food: boil and drink with sugar as a cordial when "one cannot drink coffee"
264. Encino	Quercus gambelii Nutt.	New Mexico-Spanish	Curtin, 1947	Felon on thumb: bathe in tepid tea made from bark. Sores and external cancers: boil branches apply lukewarm lotion, sprinkle with powdered bark and bandage. Malaria: boil bark, place outside overnight, drink in morning. Diarrhea: same as for malaria.
	Quercus sp.	Nueva Leon-Monterrey	Lundell, 1934	Loose teeth
265. Entraña	Opuntia arborescens Engelm.	New Mexico-Spanish	Curtin, 1947	Diuretic: make tea from flowers. Hair tonic: decoct from roots.
(Flor de Entraña)	Opuntia sp.	New Mexico-Spanish	Ford, 1966	Excessive menstruation: dry flowers, grind, and insert vaginally (3)
266. Epazote (see Pazote)				
267. Escoba de la Víbora	Gutierrezia Sarothrae	New Mexico-Spanish	Curtin, 1947 Ford, 1966	See Colláille
(see also Colláille)	Gutierrezia Sarothrae	New Mexico-Spanish	Shulman and Smith, 1962	Liniment: steep and use. Tea: steep and use

Spanish Name	Botanical Name	Location	Reference	Use
268. Escobilla	Buddleia scordioides H.B.K.	San Luís Potosí-Charcas	Whiting, 1934	Indigestion and empacho: boil in water
(Escobillo)	Buddleia scordioides H.B.K.	San Luís Potosí-Charcas	Whiting, 1934	Stomach trouble: boil in water
(Escobillo Savilla)	Buddleia scordioides	San Luís Potosí-Charcas	Lundell, 1934	Constipation and bad stomach
269. Esconcionera	unidentified	Chihuahua-Tepehuán	Pennington, 1963a	Stomach cramps: use roots to make strong tea
270. Espadaña	unidentified	Chihuahua-Tepehuán	Pennington, 1963a	Fever: make tea
271. Espanita	?Loeselia sp.	Durango-Rio Grande near La Ferreria	Riley and Trujillo, 1956	Pimples on face: boil in water and use as wash
272. Espanto Vaquero	Ipomea sp.	San Luís Potosí-Charcas	Lundell and White, 1934	Kidney and urinary troubles. Pains in shoulders.
273. Espinoncillo	Loeselia mexicana (Lam.) Brand	Valley of Mexico-Tepotzlan	Redfield, 1928	Fevers: boil leaves and take as purgative
	L. coccinea Don	Western Mexico	Rose, 1899	Fever: make tea from leaves and stems

274. Estafiate (Ajenjo, Istafiate)	<u>Artemisia</u> <u>mexicana</u> Willd.	New Mexico-Spanish	Curtin, 1947	Diarrhea and vomiting: make tea and give to babies as a purge. Stomachache: drink tea. Cough: mash plant with water, place in a rag and give to children to suck. Rheumatism: make solution for bathing.
	<u>Artemisia</u> <u>tridentata</u>	New Mexico-Spanish	Robbins, et al., 1916	Indigestion, flatulence, cough: see Chamiso Hediondo
	<u>Artemisia</u> <u>frigida</u> Willd.	New Mexico-Spanish	Jones, 1931	Stomach disorders: take infusion
(Estafiata)	<u>Artemisia</u> <u>frigida</u> Willd.	New Mexico	Wooton and Standley, 1915	
(Istafiate)	<u>A</u>. <u>ludoviciana</u> Nutt. ssp. <u>mexicana</u> (Willd.) Keck	Chihuahua-Chihuahua	Zingg, 1932	Colic: give decoction to children
(Istafiate)	<u>A</u>. <u>ludoviciana</u> Nutt.	San Luís Potosí-Charcas	Lundell, 1934	Food: toast and powder and give to babies with breast milk
	<u>Artemisia</u> sp.	New Mexico-Spanish	White, 1941	
	<u>Artemisia</u> sp. [Rocky Mt. sage]	New Mexico-Spanish	Shulman and Smith, 1962	Stomachache: take tea. Witches.

Spanish Name	Botanical Name	Location	Reference	Use
	<u>Artemisia</u> sp.	New Mexico-Spanish	Marquez, 1964	Menstrual cramping and diarrhea: see Colláile for recipe
	<u>Artemisia</u> sp.	New Mexico-Spanish	Ford, 1966	Stomachache: take as tea (3)
	<u>Artemisia</u> sp.	Chihuahua-Juarez	Ford and Ford, 1965	
	<u>Artemisia</u> sp.	Durango-Durango	Riley and Trujillo, 1956	Stomach upset:(child) grind stems, leaves and flowers, mix with milk and give; (adult) take as tea before meals and at night.
	<u>Franseria</u> <u>acanthicarpa</u>	Chihuahua-Tepehuán	Pennington, 1963a	Stomach upset: use leaves to make tea. Inflammations: crush leaves for poultice. Diarrhea: heat whole plant and sit on it.
	unidentified	San Luís Potosí-Charcas	Whiting, 1934	Fright
	unidentified	Durango-Llano Grande near La Ferreria	Riley and Trujillo, 1956	Stomachaches: boil with milk, cool and drink liquid before breakfast. Children upset by mother's milk: boil

				crumbled leaves with milk and crumbled egg shell; cool and feed to child
	unidentified	Durango-San Pedro across river from La Ferreria	Riley and Trujillo, 1956	Ulcers: boil leaves and take liquid each night for 5 days
275. Estafiate Prieto	unidentified	Chihuahua-Tarahumar	Pennington, 1963b	Intestinal upsets: use roots and stems along with 2 other unidentified plants and decoct
276. Estramonio	<u>Datura</u> sp.	New Mexico-Spanish	Curtin, 1947	See Toloache
277. Estrella	<u>Milla</u> <u>biflora</u> Cav.	New Mexico	Tidestrom and Kittell, 1941	
278. Estrella del Norte	<u>Echinocystis</u> <u>lobata</u> Torr. and Gray	New Mexico-Taos Pueblo	Curtin, 1947	Rheumatism: bake green fruit, split open and bind on afflicted members.
	<u>Asphodelus</u> <u>fistulosus</u> L.	San Luís Potosí-Charcas	Whiting, 1934	
279. Eucalita	<u>Eucaluptus</u> sp.	Nueva Leon-Monterrey	Lundell, 1934	Cough: use with other herbs
280. Flor de Alquitrán (see Alquitrán)	unidentified			

Spanish Name	Botanical Name	Location	Reference	Use
281. Flor Altea	Hibiscus syriacus	Nueva Leon-Monterrey	Lundell, 1934	Cough
282. Flor de Baraca	unidentified	Chihuahua-Parral	Riley and Trujillo, 1956	Coughs, colds, fevers: boil flowers, stems and leaves, and take every 2 hours for 3 days. (may combine with Caña Fistula for remedy for bad bronchial cough with fever)
283. Flor de Bougainbilla	Bougainvillea spectabilis	San Luís Potosí-Charcas	Lundell, 1934	Cough: drink in water
284. Flor de Camaron	Caesalpinia pulcherrima (L.) Swartz	Valley of Mexico-Tepotzlan	Redfield, 1928	Whooping cough: see Cabellito de Angel. Cough: boil with Flor de Molenillo (Malvaviscus) and armadillo shell
285. Flor de Cardo Santo (see Cardo Santo)				
286. Flor de Castilla	Rosa sp.	San Luís Potosí-Charcas	Lundell, 1934	Enema: boil and use
287. Flor de Chicascle	Wigandia kunthii Choisy	Valley of Mexico-Tepotzlan	Redfield, 1928	Abdominal pains: boil ground leaves and take

					infusion
288.	Flor de Clamaclancle	Solanum madrense Fernald	Valley of Mexico-Tepotzlan	Redfield, 1928	Vomiting in nursing baby: boil, mix with alcohol, give to mother to drink and to wash breasts
289.	Flor de un Dia	Sanvitalia ocymoides	San Luís Potosí-Charcas	Lundell, 1934	
290.	Flor de Jamica	unidentified	New Mexico-Spanish	White, 1941	
291.	Flor de Limon	Citrus aurantifolia (Christm.) Swingle	Valley of Mexico-Tepotzlan	Redfield, 1928	Fretfulness (la mohina): treat anger and ill-temper with warm drinks, e.g. lime flowers made into tea and sweetened
292.	Flor de Molenillo	Malvaviscus conzattii Greenm.	Valley of Mexico-Tepotzlan	Redfield, 1928	Cough: for recipe see Flor de Camaron
293.	Flor de Muerto	Tagetes erecta L.	Chihuahua-Chihuahua	Zingg, 1932	Diarrhea: take decoction
294.	Flor de Nacahuila	Cordia boissieri	Nueva Leon-Monterrey	Lundell, 1934	
295.	Flor de Nacahuite	Solanum fontanesianum Dunal	Valley of Mexico-Tepotzlan	Redfield, 1928	Cough: boil plant and drink tea. Restlessness during fevers: boil with Hinojo (Anethum), Flor de Tilia (Tilia), la Peonia (Peonia), Flor de

Spanish Name	Botanical Name	Location	Reference	Use
				Manita, nutmeg, cinnamon, and magnesia powder
296. Flor de Naranja (see also Azahar)	unidentified [orange tree] Citris sp.	Chihuahua-Parral	Riley and Trujillo, 1956	Insomnia: boil flowers, sweeten, take before going to bed
	unidentified	Durango-Durango	Riley and Trujillo, 1956	Nerves and heart condition: take as tea twice daily
297. Flor de Palma (also called Palma Chino)	Yucca sp.	Chihuahua-Chihuahua	Zingg, 1932	Colds: drink decoction made from flowers
	Yucca sp.	San Luís Potosí-Charcas	Lundell, 1934	Cough
298. Flor de la Paz	Nymphaea ?ampla DC	Coahuila-Torreón	Kelly, 1965	Chest cough: use with other items in tea
299. Flor de Peña	Selaginella cuspidata	Chihuahua-Tarahumar	Bennett and Zingg, 1935	Colic and indigestion. Food: use to sweeten tesguino.
(Flor de la Peña)	Selaginella ?cuspidata Link	Coahuila-Torreón	Kelly, 1965	Bilis: use in related complications; one item in a tea
	Selaginella sp.	Chihuahua-Chihuahua	Zingg, 1932	Colic and indigestion

	Selaginella sp.	San Luís Potosí-Charcas	Lundell, 1934	
300. Flor de Piedra	*Parmelia reticulata*	Chihuahua-Tepehuán	Pennington, 1963a	Venereal disease and kidney ailments: make tea, leave outside overnight, drink
301. Flor de San Diego	*Laelia* sp.	Valley of Mexico-Tepotzlan	Redfield, 1928 Field, 1953	Prevention of abortion when pregnant woman cannot satisfy a food craving. See Azucena.
302. Flor de San Juan	*Anogra runcinata* (Engelm.) Woot. and Standl.	New Mexico-Spanish	Curtin, 1947	Kidney trouble: boil flowers in water, add sugar and drink. Inflamed throat and/or tonsil trouble: make fresh flowers into paste, spread between 2 pieces of cloth, place on throat as a counter-irritant. Freckles: to "cure," rub petals on skin.

Spanish Name	Botanical Name	Location	Reference	Use
	Macrosiphonia lanuginosa (Mart. and Gal.) Hemsl.	Coahuila-Torreón	Kelly, 1965	Clearing the sight: use blossom to make decoction to drop in eye
	unidentified	Durango-Llano Grande near La Ferreria	Riley and Trujillo, 1956	Toothache: boil flowers, cool, use to rinse mouth
303. Flor de Santa Rita	Castilleja integra A. Gray C. leariaefolia	New Mexico-Spanish	Curtin, 1947	Diuretic: take sweetened tea every 2-3 hours. Inflammation of skin and leprosy: for recipe see Caña Agria.
304. Flor Sauco	Sambucus mexicana Presl	Nueva Leon-Monterrey	Lundell, 1934	Cough: use with other herbs
(Flor de Saugua)	Sambucus mexicana Presl	Coahuila-Saltillo	Lundell, 1934	Cough
(Flor de Sauz)	Sambucus mexicana Presl	New Mexico-Spanish	Curtin, 1947	Fever, Paralysis, food: see Capulín Silvestre

see Capulín Silvestre				
305. Flor de Tilia (de Bola)	*Clethra* (Prob. *mexicana* DC)	Coahuila-Torreón	Kelly, 1965	Pain in heart: palpitations, difficulty in breathing and nervousness: take decoction of several items
306. Flor de Tilia (de Estrella)	*Taonabo* sp. (Prob. *oocarpa* Rose)	Coahuila-Torreón	Kelly, 1965	Same as preceding item
	Ternstroemia Pringlei	Valley of Mexico-Tepotzlan	Field, 1953	Pneumonia, coughs, throat infections, spitting blood: boil in water until half has evaporated, add cognac, drink small glass whenever necessary.

Spanish Name	Botanical Name	Location	Reference	Use
	Tilia sp.	Valley of Mexico-Tepotzlan	Redfield, 1928	Restlessness during fevers: for recipe see Flor de Nacahuite
307. Flor de Venodillo	Swietenia humilis Zucc.	Western Mexico	Rose, 1899	Chest pains: use seeds to make tea
308. Florefundia	Datura candida	Valley of Mexico-Tepotzlan	Redfield, 1928	Toothache: see Bomba
309. Fresa	Potentilla sp. cf. exsul	Chihuahua-Tepehuan	Pennington, 1963a	Fever: use leaves to make tea
310. Fresa Cimarrona	Potentilla Thurberi	Chihuahua-Tarahumar	Pennington, 1963b	Food: eat berries
311. Fresno	Fraxinus sp.	?Sonora-Yaqui	Holden, et al., 1936	Rabies: drink tea made from leaves and bark
	Fraxinus sp.	Valley of Mexico-Tepotzlan	Redfield, 1928	Headache: mix leaves with wine and apply as poultice
312. Frijoles	Phaseolus sp.	New Mexico	Tidestrom and Kittell, 1941	Food: eat cooked
	Phaseolus sp.	New Mexico-Spanish	Shulman and Smith, 1962	Parturition: mother chews bean to facilitate afterbirth

313.	Frijolillo	*Oxytropis lambertii* Pursh	New Mexico-Spanish	Curtin, 1947	No use -- poison to animals
		Phaseolus Metcalfi	Chihuahua-Tarahumar	Pennington, 1963b	Stomach upset: see Corcomeca. Food: tesquino catalyst -- see Corcomeca.
		Erythrina flabelliformis	Chihuahua-Tarahumar	Pennington, 1963b	Toothache: see Chilocote. Intestinal disorders: see Chilocote.
314.	Fruita Amarilla	*Ulmus LeSueurii* *U. mexicana*	Chihuahua-Tarahumar	Pennington, 1963b	Food: eat in atole
315.	Garavatillo	*Mimosa biuncifera* Benth.	San Luís Potosí-Charcas	Whiting, 1934	
316.	Garbancillo	*Lupinus aduncus* Greene	New Mexico-Spanish	Curtin, 1947	Sores (running sores on children's faces): make tea from leaves to bathe sores and then apply dry, pulverized leaves
317.	Garrambullo	*Opuntia leptocaulis* DC.	New Mexico-Spanish	Wooton and Standley, 1915	
318.	Garumbullo	*Proboscidea* sp. *Martynia fragens*	Chihuahua-Tarahumar	Pennington, 1963b	Food: boil fresh leaves, drain, add to beans; eat seeds raw
319.	Gediondillo (Jediondillo)	*Bocconia arborea* S. Wats.	Valley of Mexico-Tepotzlan	Redfield, 1928 Field, 1953	Headache: plaster piece of leaf on temple with soap

Spanish Name	Botanical Name	Location	Reference	Use
320. Geranio	Pelargonium graveoleus L'Hér.	New Mexico-Spanish	Curtin, 1947	Headache: mash leaves, add salt and vinegar, bind on forehead. Earache: warm leaves and place in ear.
321. Gobernadora (Yerba Gobernadora) (see also Hediondilla)	Larrea glutinosa Engelm.	New Mexico-Spanish	Curtin, 1947	Rheumatism: rub dry, ground leaves on limbs or boil in water and bathe. Kidney trouble: take decoction of leaves. Bruises and wounds: steep leaves and twigs in boiling water and apply as poultice.
	Larrea tridentata	New Mexico-Spanish	White, 1941	
	Larrea tridentata	New Mexico-Spanish	Ford, 1966	Swelling: grind and wrap with cloth around affected area (3)
	Larrea tridentata	New Mexico-Spanish	Shulman and Smith, 1962	Cramps or rheumatic pain: grind with wild tobacco and Oshá mix with pine pitch and apply
	Larrea tridentata	Chihuahua-Juarez	Ford and Ford, 1965	Stomach: use for bad stomach

(Wame Gobernadora)	*Larrea tridentata* (DC.) Coville	Chihuahua-Chihuahua	Zingg, 1932	Rheumatism: fry leaves and use as hot poultice
	Larrea tridentata	San Luís Potosí-Charcas	Whiting, 1934	Stomach trouble: boil and drink
	Larrea tridentata	Nueva Leon-Monterrey	Lundell, 1934	
	L. divaricata Cav.	Coahuila-Torreón	Kelly, 1965	Abdominal pain: boil and drink. Rheumatism: apply externally.
	L. divaricata Cav.	Baja California-Paipai	Owen, 1963	Frío: for recipe see Yerba del Pasmo
	L. tridentata *Covillea tridentata* (DC.) Vail	Western Mexico	Rose, 1899	Pains in the womb: take tea made from leaves and branches. Rheumatism: fry leaves and twigs in tallow and apply as hot poultice.
322. Golondrina (La) (see also Yerba de la Golondrina)	*Euphorbia* sp.	New Mexico-Cochiti	Lange, 1959	Sores, burns, cuts: apply ground plant
	Euphorbia sp.	Arizona	Kearney and Peebles, 1964	Snakebite
	Euphorbia sp.	?Sonora-Yaqui	Holden, et al., 1936	Snakebite: mash to pulp and apply paste. Rabies: apply to bite and steep

Spanish Name	Botanical Name	Location	Reference	Use
				in water and drink liquid.
	<u>Euphorbia</u> sp.	Sonora-Opata	Hrdlicka, 1904	Snakebite
	<u>E. melanadenia</u> Torr.	Baja California-Paipai	Owen, 1963	Rattlesnake bite: boil whole plant, drink tea and use as wash
	<u>Euphorbia</u> sp.	San Luís Potosí-Charcas	Lundell, 1934	Medicinal
	<u>Euphorbia</u> sp.	Nueva Leon-Monterrey	Lundell, 1934	
	<u>Richmondra argentea</u> H.B.K.	San Luís Potosí-Charcas	Whiting, 1934	Stomach pains: boil in water and take
	<u>Dichondra argentea</u> H.B.K.	San Luís Potosí-Charcas	Whiting, 1934	Same as preceding item
323. Goma de Sonora	<u>Larrea tridentata</u> (DC.) Coville [lac insect host plant]	Sonora-Yaqui	Holden, et al., 1936	Dysentery: boil 3 sticks of gum, add Anís, cinnamon, and essence of mint; strain and add alcohol as preservative; drink 3 times a day
324. Goma de Trementina	unidentified	New Mexico-Spanish	Ford, 1966	See Trementina

325. Gomilla (Gomea)	*Courseta glandulosa* Gray [host plant of lac insect]	Arizona-Spanish	Toumey, 1895	Lungs and stomach troubles
326. Gordolobo	*Verbascum thapsus* L.	California-Spanish	Curtin, 1947	This is California name for this plant. Pulmonary diseases and sprains: use externally.
(Yerba Gordolobo)	unidentified	New Mexico-Spanish	White, 1941	
	Gnaphalium Maccounii	Chihuahua-Tepehuán	Pennington, 1963a	Heart pains: take tea made from leaves. Coughing spells: use tea made from leaves and flowers.
	G. cf. *canescens* DC.	Coahuila-Torreón	Kelly, 1965	Chest cough (especially early tuberculosis): take decoction with other ingredients
	G. semiamplexicaule	San Luís Potosí-Charcas	Lundell, 1934	Cough: make gargle
327. Gordo Lobo (Manzanilla del Rio)	unidentified	Chihuahua-Parral	Riley and Trujillo, 1956	Pulmonary inflammation and cough: boil flower and stems and take 3 times a day for 9 days or until cured

Spanish Name	Botanical Name	Location	Reference	Use
	unidentified	Zacatecas-Zacatecas	Riley and Trujillo, 1956	Coughs: boil in water, take tea before meals for 9 days. Venereal disease and urinary infections: boil and take twice daily for 9 days.
328. Gordo del Sapo	unidentified	Zacatecas-Zacatecas	Riley and Trujillo, 1956	Coughs and venereal disease: boil and take
329. Grama China	_Hilaria_ sp.? or _Paspalum_	Zacatecas-Zacatecas	Riley and Trujillo, 1956	Kidney and urinary dieseases: boil roots; take infusion twice daily for 9 days
330. Granada (see also Cáscara de Granada)	_Punica granatum_ L.	Valley of Mexico-Tepotzlan	Redfield, 1928	Whiteness of lips (rotten mouth): use leaves with guayaba (_Psidium guajaba_ L.), roast, grind and make into infusion to use as wash
(Granada Agu)	_Punica granatum_	Zacatecas-Zacatecas	Riley and Trujillo, 1956	Dysentery and inflammations of female genitals: grind fruit with water and drink before meals
331. Grangene	_Ephedra aspera_ Engelm.	San Luís Potosí-Charcas	Whiting, 1934	

332. Granjén	Celtis pallida Torr.	Coahuila-Torreón	Kelly, 1965	Food: see Capulín
333. Guaccimas	Guazuma ulmifolia	San Luís Potosí-Charcas	Lundell, 1934	Urinary disorders: boil with other herbs
334. Guácima	unidentified	Chihuahua-Parral (from Oaxaca)	Riley and Trujillo, 1956	Kidney troubles; back-aches, veneral disease: boil 1 seed in water and take 3 times a day for 9 days
335. Guachichile (Huichichili)	Loeselia coccinea Brand	Chihuahua-Juarez	Jones, 1932	Fever and colds: use plant to make tea; drink and bathe
	Loeselia sp.	Chihuahua-Tepehuán	Pennington, 1963a	Chest pains: take strong tea
	L. coccinea Brand	San Luís Potosí-Charcas	Lundell, 1934	
	L. coccinea Brand	Nueva Leon-Monterrey	Lundell, 1934	
	unidentified	Chihuahua-Tepehuán	Pennington, 1963a	Fever: use to make tea
336. Guachi-chiligo	Loeselia coerulea Don	San Luís Potosí-Charcas	Lundell, 1934	
337. Guácia	unidentified	Zacatecas-Zacatecas	Riley and Trujillo, 1956	Fits: boil limb of tree in water and take liquid each a.m.

Spanish Name	Botanical Name	Location	Reference	Use
				for 9 days
338. Guaco	_Cleome serrulata_ Pursh	New Mexico-Spanish	Curtin, 1947	Inflammation from poisonous insects: crush leaves and apply. Anemia: boil flowers in water with nail; drink strained decoction cold. Stomach trouble: boil 3 hours with corn and cloves and eat greens. "Gripes" in the intestines: mash leaves with Añil del Muerto, mix with hot water, strain and drink. Food: eat seeds and greens.
	Mikania guaco H. et B.	Mexico	Martinez, 1959	
339. Guadalupe	_Lobelia laxiflora_	Chihuahua-Tepehuán	Pennington, 1963a	Toothache: place leaf between cheek and gums.
340. Guaje Cirial	_Crescentia alota_	Zacatecas-Zacatecas	Riley and Trujillo, 1956	Bronchial troubles and coughs: boil part of a fruit (seeds, pith and rind) and take liquid twice daily for 5 days
341. Guajillo	_Cassia laevigata_ Willd.	Valley of Mexico-Tepotzlan	Redfield, 1928	Respiratory troubles (Nahuatl name = "wind

				machine") grind plant and place in alcohol with Jarilla (*Senecio*) rub infusion on chest
342. Guamúchil	*Pithecellobium dulce*	Chihuahua-Tarahumar	Pennington, 1963b	Food: eat fruit; add arils to tortilla dough. Dye: rust color. Tanning.
343. Guásima	*Guazuma ulmifolia*	Chihuahua-Tarahumar	Pennington, 1963b	Food: grind seeds, make into cakes, bake; use to make beverage.
	Guazuma ulmifolia	Chihuahua-Tepehuán	Pennington, 1963a	Shortness of breath: boil bark and drink liquid
	unidentified	Zacatecas-Zacatecas	Riley and Trujillo, 1956	Venereal disease or urinary trouble: grind nuts (seeds) into water strain, beat, restrain, take daily for 9 days
344. Guata	*Juniperus californica* Carr.	Baja California-Paipai	Owen, 1963	Pains in bones, muscles, and members: strip off inner bark, tie into small packet, pour boiling water over it, steep, when red, use as liniment.
345. Guatamote	*Baccharis glutinosa* Pers.	Baja California-Kiliwa	Meigs, 1939	Boils: heat leaves and apply externally

Spanish Name	Botanical Name	Location	Reference	Use
346. Guayaba	*Psidium guajava*	Chihuahua-Tarahumar	Bennett and Zingg, 1935	Food: eat fruit raw
	Psidium guajava	Valley of Mexico-Tepotzlan	Redfield, 1928	Whiteness of lips: for recipe see Granada
347. Guayabillo	*Eriosema grandiflorum* (S. and C.) Seem.	Valley of Mexico-Tepotzlan	Redfield, 1928	Sore feet: wash with infusion of leaves
348. Guayes	unidentified	New Mexico-Spanish	Shulman and Smith, 1962	Venereal disease: boil use to wash sores. Colds: use as tea.
349. Gueso de Mamell	*Pithecoctenium echinatum* Schl.	San Luís Potosí-Charcas	Lundell, 1934	Hair dressing: (to curl hair) grind, beat vigorously and rub in hair
350. Guirote de Culebra	*Serjania mexicana*	Chihuahua-Tarahumar	Pennington, 1963b	Bruises, etc.: see Diente de Culebra
351. Guirote de Leche	unidentified	Chihuahua-Tarahumar	Pennington, 1963b	Insect bites: apply milky excrescence on stems. Sprains: apply milky excrescence as salve.
352. Habas	*Vicia faba* L.	New Mexico-Spanish	Curtin, 1947	Food: eat as beans. Pneumonia (to prevent) and counteract "cold on lungs": brown in oven, boil, salt, and

					drink as soup. Pneumonia: apply paste of ground beans and hot water to chest and back. Soreness in mouth: apply ground beans.
353.	Harta Reina	Piqueria trinervia Cav.	Valley of Mexico-Tepotzlan	Redfield, 1928	Los aires and fever: see Alta Reina
354.	Hediondilla (see Gobernadora)	Larrea glutinosa Engelm.	New Mexico-Spanish	Curtin, 1947	Rheumatism, kidney trouble, bruises and wounds: see Gobernadora
		Larrea tridentata (DC.) Coville	Chihuahua-Juarez	Ford and Ford, 1965	Stomach: use for bad stomach (8)
	(Hediondia)	Larrea tridentata (DC.) Coville	Arizona-Sonora-Papago, Mexican	Lumholtz, 1912	Wounds. Gastric disturbance: take internally.
355.	Higos	Ficus Carica L.	New Mexico-Spanish	Curtin, 1947	Laxative: eat fruit. Asthma: smoke dry leaves in pipe, inhale deeply. Ruptured navel in newborn: apply cut-open fig.
356.	Higuera	Ficus radulina	Chihuahua-Tarahumar	Bennett and Zingg, 1935	Food: cook young leaves in water to make a beverage or add salt for a sauce to eat with chile

Spanish Name	Botanical Name	Location	Reference	Use
				eat fruit raw
	<u>Ricinus</u> <u>communis</u>	Chihuahua-Tarahumar	Bennett and Zingg, 1935	Headache: wrap leaves in cloth around head. Sores (running): make salve by mixing leaves with lard and cook (wrapped in leaves) in ashes
(Higueria)	<u>Ricinus</u> <u>communis</u>	Baja California-Paipai	Owen, 1963	Skin eruptions and boils: crush ripe seed and use oil on irritation
(Higuerilla)	<u>Ricinus</u> <u>communis</u>	Chihuahua-Tepehuán	Pennington, 1963a	Goitres or inflammations: use leaves to make poultice. Purgative: use crushed seeds.
(Hineldo)	<u>Anethum</u> <u>graveolens</u> L.	New Mexico-Spanish	White, 1941	
(Neldo)	<u>Anethum</u> <u>graveolens</u> L.	San Luís Potosí-Charcas	Lundell, 1934	
357. Hinojo	<u>Foeniculum</u> <u>vulgare</u> Hill [fennel]	New Mexico-Spanish	Curtin, 1947	Heart trouble: boil seeds in water, add gold leaf and drink 3 times a day. Post-parturition (to clear system after childbirth): chew seeds or drink tea

				made from dry plant. Female trouble (for young girls who suffer from a lapse of catamenia) chew and swallow leaves.
	[fennel]	New Mexico-Spanish	Shulman and Smith, 1962	Cramps: use for gas in stomach
	<u>Anethum</u> <u>graveolens</u> L.	New Mexico-Spanish	Ford, 1966	Food: use to make pickles (3)
	<u>Anethum</u> <u>graveolens</u> L.	Chihuahua-Juarez	Ford and Ford, 1965	Tea (8)
	<u>Anethum</u> <u>graveolens</u> L. [dill]	Valley of Mexico-Tepotzlan	Redfield, 1928	Restlessness during fevers: for recipe see Flor de Nacahuite.
	unidentified	San Luís Potosí-Charcas	Lundell, 1934	To cause sweating: use with other herbs
358. Hinseseli	<u>Loeselia</u> sp.	Western Mexico	Rose, 1899	Fever and ague: take tea made from leaves. Purgative: take cold infusion.
359. Hipazote (see Pazote)				
360. Hoja de babisa	<u>Anemopsis</u> <u>californica</u>	Chihuahua-Chihuahua	Zingg, 1932	Sores and boils: see Bavisa

Spanish Name	Botanical Name	Location	Reference	Use
361. Hoja de Boldo	unidentified	Chihuahua-Parral	Riley and Trujillo, 1956	Inflammation of the liver: boil leaves and drink each a.m. before eating until cured
362. Hoja Cena	unidentified	Baja California-Paipai	Owen, 1963	Menstrual difficulties: grind root and boil in water; drink in place of water during menstrual period
363. Hoja de Sen	<u>Cassia</u> sp.	Chihuahua-Parral (from Oaxaca)	Riley and Trujillo, 1956	Purgative: boil dry leaves, take as needed
364. Hojas de Nogal (see also Nogal)	<u>Juglans</u> sp.	San Luís Potosí-Charcas	Lundell, 1934	Blood (to increase or give strength)
365. Hojasen	<u>Flourensia</u> <u>cernua</u> DC.	Chihuahua-Chihuahua	Zingg, 1932	Purgative: take decoction
	<u>Flourensia</u> <u>cernua</u> DC.	Mexico	Martinez, 1959	
366. Hongos	Fungus	New Mexico-Tewa	Robbins, et al., 1916	Food: cook and eat
	Fungus	New Mexico-Spanish	Curtin, 1947	Broken eardrum: powder puff-balls and place in ear with cotton.

				Wounds (to stop bleeding): sprinkle with dry powder.
367. Huachalalá Palo de	unidentified	Zacatecas-Zacatecas	Riley and Trujillo, 1956	Bronchial diseases and coughs: boil bark and take liquid 3 times a day for 2-3 days
368. Huacha-laláte	unidentified	Zacatecas-Zacatecas	Riley and Trujillo, 1956	Stomach ulcers: take decoction of bark (boiled with water) daily for several days. Kidney infections: take decoction in a.m.
369. Huachi-chile	*Loeselia* sp.	Durango-Durango	Riley and Trujillo, 1956	Fever (especially scar-let): grind stems and leaves with water and bathe daily for 2-3 days
	unidentified	Durango-Llano Grande near La Ferreria	Riley and Trujillo, 1956	Fevers: boil, sweeten and drink
370. Huaco (Itamor-real)	*Aristolochia* sp.	Zacatecas-Zacatecas	Riley and Trujillo, 1956	Snake and scorpion bites: boil a piece of vine in water and take twice daily for 4-5 days
371. Huaspór	unidentified	Durango-Llano Grande near La Ferreria	Riley and Trujillo, 1956	Body sores: use lower stems and roots to make a wash to bathe body.

Spanish Name	Botanical Name	Location	Reference	Use
				Tranquilizer: as bath?
372. Hueso de Cereza	*Prunus cerasus* L.	New Mexico-Spanish	Curtin, 1947	Kidney trouble: boil cherry pits to make tea
373. Hueso de Mamey	*Calocarpum mammosum* *Mammea americana* L.	Valley of Mexico-Tepotzlan	Field, 1953 Redfield, 1928	Cathartic compound: grind stone and use with other ingredients
374. Huichichili	*Loeselia coccinea* Brand	Chihuahua-Juarez	Jones, 1932	Fever and colds: see Guachichile
375. Huinecastle	*Enterolobium cyclocarpum* Griseb.	Western Mexico	Rose, 1899	Colds: use bark to make sweet syrup. Soap and tanning: use bark.
376. Huisache	*Acacia* sp.	Sonora-Yaqui	Holden, et al., 1936	Headache: make pulp of bark, moisten with male urine and apply as a poultice to head
	A. farnesiana (L.) Willd.	San Luís Potosí-Charcas	Whiting, 1934	Use to make ink for writing
377. Igualamo (Jari)	*Vitex mollis*	Chihuahua-Tarahumar	Pennington, 1963b	Fever: steep leaves
378. Incienso	*Encelia farinosa* Gray	California ?	Beal, 1943	Incense: burn gum

				Medicinal use: smear on body.
	Encelia farinosa Gray	Arizona and Baja	Kearney and Peebles, 1964	Gum: chew gum. Incense: burn gum as incense in churches (Baja).
379. Indio	*Aristolochia aguicida* *A. foetida*	Northeastern Mexico	Lundell, 1934	
380. Ineldo (Neldo)	*Anethum graveolens* [dill]	Nueva Leon-Monterrey	Lundell, 1934	
381. Inmortal	*Asclepiodora decumbens* Nutt.	New Mexico-Spanish	Van der Eerden, 1948	Laxative (especially for pregnant women): take powdered root with Yerba del Lobo (*Helenium*) and brandy or whiskey
		New Mexico-Spanish	Curtin, 1947	Back and neck pains from fever: use ground root in poultice with water and whiskey. Labor pains: take ground root in cold water and also, rub on abdomen. Expulsion of afterbirth: drink hot decoction of powdered root. Asthma or shortness of breath: take tea every hour or so.

Spanish Name	Botanical Name	Location	Reference	Use
				Catarrh: place ground root in nose to cause sneezing.
	Asclepias sp.? [spider milkweed]	New Mexico-Spanish	Shulman and Smith, 1962	All ailments: "almost foolproof", use whenever you feel ill as tea. Tuberculosis: tea. Headaches: grind and sniff. Cold, sinus headache, to prevent colds: tea. Shoulder pain: use tea. Fever: use tea.
	Asclepias capricornu Woodson	New Mexico-Spanish	Ford, 1966	Cuts: grind root and apply (4). Nosebleed: grind root and inhale (3). Internal bruises: take as tea (3). Head cold: grind and place on nose with salt to cause sneezing (3).
	Asclepias tuberosa	Chihuahua-Tarahumar	Pennington, 1963b	Nasal obstruction: sniff dry, pulverized stems
382. Inojo, Semilla de	unidentified	Zacatecas-Zacatecas	Riley and Trujillo, 1956	Intestinal flu and dysentery: boil seeds and take after meals

383. Ipasote or Ipazote (see Pazote)				
384. Islaya	Prunus ilicifolia (Nutt.) Walp.	Baja California-Paipai	Owen, 1963	Colds: drink tea made from leaves
385. Istafiate (see Estafiate)				
386. Itamo Real	Pellaea cordata	Valley of Mexico-Tepepan	Madsen, 1965	Cough (caused by cold): take tea -- see Caña de Castilla
	Ephedra aspera Engelm.	San Luís Potosí-Charcas	Lundell, 1934	Bladder trouble: boil with other herbs
387. Ixpule	Pinaropappus roseus	Valley of Mexico-Tepepan	Madsen, 1965	Dysentery (with white stools, caused by cold): take tea
388. Jaboncillo	Sapindus Saponaria L. var. Drummondii (Hook. and Arn.)	New Mexico-Spanish	Wooton and Standley, 1915 Kearney and Peebles, 1964	Washing: use fruits for soap in washing clothes
389. Jaltomate	Saracha jaltomata	Chihuahua-Tarahumar	Pennington, 1963b	Food: eat berries
390. Jara	Salix argophylla Nutt.	New Mexico-Tewa	Robbins, et al., 1916	No medicinal or food use given

Spanish Name	Botanical Name	Location	Reference	Use
	Salix sp.	New Mexico-Spanish	Ford, 1966	To tighten teeth: use roots (3)
391. Jari (Igualamo)	_Vitex mollis_	Chihuahua-Tarahumar	Pennington, 1963b	Food: eat fruit raw or cooked. Fever: see Igualamo.
392. Jarilla	?_Dodonaea_ sp.	Durango-Llano Grande near La Ferreria	Riley and Trujillo, 1956	Stomach upsets: grind leaves and tops of stalks with alcohol to make a paste; place on stomach and leave until dry
393. Jarillo	_Senecio salignus_ DC.	Valley of Mexico-Tepotzlan	Redfield, 1928	Respiratory diseases: for recipe see Guajillo
	Selloa glutinosa	Valley of Mex-Tepepan	Madsen, 1965	Anger sickness (treated by curandero de aire): massage body and apply stomach poultice of this plant dipped in alcohol. Also, drink rue tea.
394. Jarillo de Río	_Baccharis glutinosa_	Chihuahua-Tarahumar	Pennington, 1963b	Skin infections: bruise young leaves and apply as poultice
	unidentified	Chihuahua-Tepehuán	Pennington, 1963a	Infertility in cows: cook leaves and feed to cow
395. Jarita	_Salix exigua_ Nutt.	New Mexico-Spanish	Curtin, 1947	Pyorrhoea: boil bark for tea

396. Jaronsillo or Javonsillo	*Parosela caudata* Rydb.	San Luís Potosí-Charcas	Whiting, 1934	
397. Jícama	*Exogonium bracteatum*	Chihuahua-Tarahumar	Pennington, 1963b	Food: eat young roots raw; older roots, pound, heat and eat with pinole or atole
398. Jicona	unidentified	Durango-Llano Grande near La Ferreria	Riley and Trujillo, 1956	Heart trouble: shred leaves and mix with hog's lard and spread on chest as a poultice; apply twice daily for 6 days
399. Jitomate	*Lycopersicum esculentum* Mill. *Solanum lycopersicum* L.	Valley of Mexico-Tepotzlan	Redfield, 1928	Granular eruptions: apply infusion made of tomato leaves
400. Jocoyol	*Oxalis violacea* L.	New Mexico-Spanish	Curtin, 1947	Food: see Chocoyle. Vermifuge: see Chocoyle.
401. Juanita	*Helianthemum glomeratum*	Chihuahua-Tepehuán	Pennington, 1963a	Diarrhea: take tea made from stems
402. Juatamote	*Baccharis glutinosa* Pers.	Baja California-Paipai	Owen, 1963	Wounds, bruises, aches, pains: heat leaves over fire and apply to affected area
403. Judica	unidentified	San Luís Potosí-Charcas	Lundell, 1934	To cause sweating: use for bath. Wounds: fry in grease and apply.

Spanish Name	Botanical Name	Location	Reference	Use
404. Junco	unidentified [small cactus]	Chihuahua-Tepehuan	Pennington, 1963a	Stomach cramps: take tea made from stalk
405. Kokolmíka	_Piper_ sp.	Chihuahua-Tarahumar	Bennett and Zingg, 1935	Rheumatism: cook in water and use as bath. Arm pains: use stem as cane.
406. Laceta (Aceitilla)	_Bidens leucantha_ (L.) Willd.	Valley of Mexico-Tepotzlan	Redfield, 1928 Field, 1953	Eye trouble: see Aceitilla
407. Lama del Agua	Algae	New Mexico-Spanish	Curtin, 1947	Nosebleed: put fresh moss on back of neck and leave until it turns yellow
408. Lampaquate	_Gnaphalium_ sp.	Chihuahua-Tarahumar	Bennett and Zingg, 1935	Colds: boil flowers and stems and give decoction to children
409. Lantejilla	_Lepidium densiflorum_ Schrad.	Valley of Mexico-Tepotzlan	Redfield, 1928	Colds: steep in alcohol and place on chest
410. Lantén	_Plantago major_ L.	New Mexico-Spanish	Curtin, 1947	Headache: crush green leaves, add salt and bind to head
	Plantago major L.	Chihuahua-Juarez	Jones, 1932	Cuts: apply as poultice

	Plantago major L.	Chihuahua-Tarahumar	Pennington, 1963b	Constipation: take as tea
	Plantago major L.	Chihuahua-Tepehuán	Pennington, 1963a	Fever: crush roots, boil, strain, take as warm tea
	Plantago major L.	San Luís Potosí-Charcas	Lundell, 1934	Constipation
(Lantena)	*Plantago major* L.	Baja California-Paipai	Owen, 1963	Headache: bind leaves on forehead. Bruises and wounds: heat leaves and apply.
411. Lantén cimarrón	*Mimulus guttatus*	Chihuahua-Tarahumar	Pennington, 1963b	Food: eat leaves cooked with beans
412. Laurel	*Nerium Oleander* L.	New Mexico-Spanish	Curtin, 1947	Headache or neuralgia: grind dry leaf and rub on afflicted parts
	?unidentified or *Litsea*	New Mexico-Spanish	Curtin, 1947	(real Laurel from store) Fever: take tea from leaves. Food: use for seasoning.
	Litsea glaucescens H.B.K.	Western Mexico	Rose, 1899	Colds: take tea made from leaves. Food: use for seasoning.
	Litsea glaucescens H.B.K.	Chihuahua-Chihuahua	Zingg, 1932	Food: make tea and drink with sugar. Stomach gas: drink tea.

Spanish Name	Botanical Name	Location	Reference	Use
	L. pringlei Bartlett	San Luís Potosí-Charcas	Lundell, 1934	Medicinal
413. Laurel-illo	Persea americana	Chihuahua-Tepehuan	Pennington, 1963a	Diarrhea, aching gums, goitre, and wounds: see Aguacate
414. Leche de Cabra	not a plant -- goat's milk	New Mexico-Spanish	Shulman and Smith, 1962	Tuberculosis. Blood: good for blood. Ulcers: use to prevent.
415. Lecheros	Asclepias speciosa Torr.	New Mexico-Spanish	Curtin, 1947	Food: add young leaves and pods to meat dishes.
		New Mexico-Tewa	Curtin, 1947	Lactation (if faulty): take decoction. Sore breasts: take infusion of whole plant.
416. Lechona	Asclepias mexicana Cav.	Coahuila-Torreon	Kelly, 1965	Skin infection (em-peine): apply sap around edges to pre-vent spreading
417. Lechones	Asclepias galioides H.B.K.	New Mexico-Spanish	Curtin, 1947	Food: eat inside of green pods. Facial pains (to draw sore-ness out): apply milk from the plant.
	A. latifolia (Torr.) Raf.	New Mexico-Spanish	Curtin, 1947	Gum: cut stems into several segments and place in sun so that

				balls of fluid appear at ends: dry these and chew. Sores: apply fresh sap. Warts: apply fresh sap. Complexion balm: apply fresh sap.
418. Lechuguilla	*Abronia fragans* Nutt.	New Mexico-Spanish	Curtin, 1947	Lacteal stimulant: grind dry plant, boil in water to obtain syrup; strain and drink every 3rd morning before breakfast. Also, use to bathe breasts.
	Apocynum cannabinum lividum A. Nels.	New Mexico-Spanish	Curtin, 1947	Gum: made as described above for Lechones (*Asclepias latifolia*)
	Agave lechuguilla Torr.	New Mexico	Wooton and Standley, 1915	
	Senecio sp. cf. *aceinella*	Chihuahua-Tepehuan	Pennington, 1963a	Heart stimulant: take tea made from leaves
	Senecio sp.	Valley of Mexico-Tepotzlan	Redfield, 1928	Constipation or indigestion in children: boil with Hueso de Mamey, Palo Amarillo (*Tecoma stans*), and *Sacasili* (?) and give infusion

Spanish Name	Botanical Name	Location	Reference	Use
	Hieracium sp.	Western Mexico	Rose, 1899	Sores and skin diseases: use infusion of green plant as a wash or apply as powder
419. Lechuguilla Mansa	Agave perplexans Trelease	San Luís Potosí-Charcas	Whiting, 1934	Washing clothes: use root for soap
420. Lechuguilla de la Sierra	Senecio sp.	Chihuahua-Tepehuán	Pennington, 1963a	Chest pains: crush leaves and add to a tea of Vinola (Acacia cochilicantha) leaves and drink. Difficult urination: same tea as above.
421. Lechuvilla	Hieracum sp.	Durango-Rincon Grande de Magayál (3 km from La Ferreria)	Riley and Trujillo, 1956	Insect bites and sores: pulverize and moisten leaves and apply
422. Lemita	Rhus trilobata Nutt.	New Mexico-Spanish	Curtin, 1947	Food: eat berries; grind into bread; use to make beverage. Dye: black, from leaves and twigs. Hair rinse: decoct roots and rinse hair to promote growth.
	Rhus trilobata	New Mexico-Tewa	Robbins, et al., 1916	Sore mouth: grind dry bark to powder and rub on. Gum: from bush,

				chew.
423. Lengua de Buey	Family <u>Compositae</u>	Chihuahua-Tarahumar	Bennett and Zingg, 1935	Headache: heat large bundle of leaves and apply to head as poultice. Colic: apply poultice to stomach.
424. Lengua de Cervo	<u>Polypodium</u> <u>lanceolatum</u> L.	Western Mexico	Rose, 1899	Itch: use fronds to make tea
425. Lengua de Pajare	<u>Polypodium</u> <u>aviculare</u> L.	New Mexico	Tidestrom and Kittell, 1941	
426. Lengua de Perico	unidentified	Chihuahua-Tarahumar	Pennington, 1963b	Sores: heat leaves and apply as poultice
427. Lengua de Vaca	<u>Rumex</u> <u>crispus</u> L.	New Mexico-Spanish	Curtin, 1947	Food: eat leaves as greens. Headache: mash leaves with salt; bind to head. Pyorrhea: chew roots.
	<u>Rumex</u> <u>mexicanus</u> Meisn.	New Mexico	Tidestrom and Kittel, 1941	
	<u>Rumex</u> <u>mexicanus</u> Meisn.	San Luís Potosí-Charcas	Whiting, 1934	
	<u>Buddleia</u> <u>sessiliflora</u> H.B.K.	Valley of Mexico-Tepotzlan	Redfield, 1928	Fever: apply leaves to chest. Toothache: mix leaves with suet, apply to gums. Cooking: use to prepare comal.

Spanish Name	Botanical Name	Location	Reference	Use
	unidentified	Valley of Mexico-Tepotzlan	Field, 1953	Fevers, lung trouble: pulverize and apply on back over kidneys. Tumors, sores, and boils: apply paste.
	unidentified	Durango-Rincon Grande de Magayal (3 km from La Ferreria)	Riley and Trujillo, 1956	Infections of fingernail: boil branches with leaves and place finger in hot liquid 3 times; do this several times a day for 8 days
(Chile de Pajaro)	unidentified	Durango-La Ferreria	Riley and Trujillo, 1956	Dysentery: boil in water, take cup before breakfast every morning for 9 days or until relief is obtained (can mix with Yerba de Pajaro and Masarquite)
428. Lentajilla	<u>Lepidium</u> <u>virginicum</u>	Chihuahua-Tepehuán	Pennington, 1963a	Food (for sick): use seeds to make atole. Fever: make tea from stems.
429. Lentejilla (Lentajilla de Agua)	<u>Lemna</u> sp.	New Mexico	Tidestrom and Kittell, 1941	

430. Limón	Citrus limonia Osbeck.	Chihuahua-Chihuahua	Zingg, 1932	Poultice: use lemon peel; grind with avocado seed and apply warm
(see also Flor de Limón	Citrus sp.	New Mexico-Spanish	Shulman and Smith, 1962	Tuberculosis. Colds and Fevers. Liver: "good for liver" with salt.
431. Limoncillo	Pectis angustifolia Torr.	New Mexico-Spanish	Curtin, 1947	Stomach pains: make tea from whole plant
	Dyssodia pentachaeta (DC.) Robinson	San Luís Potosí-Charcas	Lundell, 1934	Constipation
432. Lina	Gilia longiflora (Torr.) G. Don	New Mexico-Tewa	Robbins, et al., 1916	Headache: grind dry flowers and leaves, mix with water and apply. Sores: use as for headache.
433. Linasa (also Linaza)	Linum lewisii Pursh	New Mexico-Spanish	Curtin, 1947	Inflammations: use linseed for poultice. Wounds (infected), swellings, mumps: grind dry seeds, mix with cornmeal, make paste with boiling water. Boils and sore throat: as above, or grind seed and mix with water or vinegar for poultice.

Spanish Name	Botanical Name	Location	Reference	Use
	Linum lewisii Pursh	New Mexico-Spanish	Ford, 1966	Wave set (4). Ulcers (4).
434. Lirio	Family Iridaceae ?Iris sp.	New Mexico-Spanish	Curtin, 1947	Smallpox: slice roots, thread on a cord and tie as necklace around throat
435. Lúpulo	Humulus Lupulus [hops?]	New Mexico-Spanish	Ford, 1966	
436. Macuchi	Nicotiana tabacum	Chihuahua-Tarahumar	Bennett and Zingg, 1935	Ceremonial smoking; incense; insect and snake repellent
437. Madroño	Arbutus arizonica Arbutus glandulosa Arbutus xalapensis	Chihuahua-Tarahumar	Pennington, 1963b	Food: eat flowers and fruits; and use to make a tesguino
438. Maiz, Flor de	Zea mays	New Mexico-Spanish	Shulman and Smith, 1962	Asthma: take tea three times per day
439. Maiz, Avena de (see also Atole)	Zea mays	New Mexico-Spanish	Shulman and Smith, 1962	Lung hemorrhage: eat (ground)
440. Majahui	Croton sp.	Chihuahua-Tarahumar	Bennett and Zingg, 1935	Paint (whitewash): pound bark and mix with lime
441. Majorana	Lantana sp.	Western Mexico	Rose, 1899	Indigestion

442. Mal de ojos	_Sphaeralcea_ sp.	Arizona-Pima	Kearney and Peebles, 1964	Sore eyes
443. Mala mujer	_Solanum rostratum_	San Luís Potosí-Charcas	Lundell, 1934	
	Cnidoscolus angusti-deus Torr.	Arizona	Kearney and Peebles, 1964	
444. Malva(s)	_Malva parviflora_ L.	New Mexico-Spanish	Van Der Eerden, 1948	Post-partum abdominal pains: boil in water with raisins and manzan-illa and take as tea
(also Malva del Campo)	_Malva parviflora_ L.	New Mexico-Spanish	Curtin, 1947	Pimples: make tea from leaves and use as a wash. Fever: take de-coction of leaves to cause sweating. Head-ache: mash leaves with salt and vinegar and place on temples. Pneumonia: tea? Em-menagogue: tea? Swol-len glands: blow dry, powdered leaves into throat. Post-partum "cleaning out of system": take as tea.
	Malva sp.? [mallow]	New Mexico-Spanish	Shulman and Smith, 1962	Rash on baby's buttocks: use in solution. Par-turition: use to expe-dite expulsion of after-

Spanish Name	Botanical Name	Location	Reference	Use
				birth.
	Malva sp.	New Mexico-Spanish	Ford, 1966	Menstrual or post-partum hemorrhaging: take tea with raisins (3)
	Malva sp.?	Chihuahua-Juarez	Ford and Ford, 1965	Stomach: good for stomach (8)
	Malva parviflora L.	Chihuahua-Chihuahua	Zingg, 1932	Douche: use decoction
	Sida rhombifolia _Abutilon trisculcatum_	Chihuahua-Tarahumar	Bennett and Zingg, 1935	Hairwash: mix juice from pounded leaves with water and use. Good for growth and gloss.
	Sida cordifolia	Chihuahua-Tepehuán	Pennington, 1963a	Purgative: take strong tea
	Malvaviscus aboreus	Chihuahua-Tepehuán	Pennington, 1963a	Fever
	Malva rotundifolia	Chihuahua-Tepehuán	Pennington, 1963a	Fever: use whole plant
	Malva parviflora L.	Valley of Mexico-Tepotzlan	Redfield, 1928	Fever: for recipe see Alta Reina

	unidentified	San Luís Potosí-Charcas	Whiting, 1934	Wounds: boil in water and use to wash
(Malvas)	unidentified	Durango-San Pedro across river from La Ferreria	Riley and Trujillo, 1956	Headaches and stomach sickness in children: grind plant and mix with mustard, vinegar, lime juice and carbonate (carbonate?); apply as poultice to head or chest and cover with a thin cloth
445. Malva de Castilla	*Malva crispa* L.	New Mexico-Spanish	Curtin, 1947	Measles: drink hot decoction of leaves. Hoarse throat: same as above. Boils and bruises: use leaves for poultice. Enema (for women): use tea with salt. Post-partum pains: take decoction of dry malva, water (boil), raisins and tequesquite.
446. Mangle	*Rhus ovata* Watts.	Baja California-Paipai	Owen, 1963	"Birth"
447. Manto de la Vergen	unidentified	Durango-La Ferreria	Riley and Trujillo, 1956	Chills and fever: boil whole dry plant and drink
448. Manzana	[apples]	Chihuahua-Tarahumar	Bennett and Zingg, 1935	

Spanish Name	Botanical Name	Location	Reference	Use
449. Manzanilla	<u>Matricaria</u> <u>Chamomilla</u> L.	New Mexico-Spanish	Van der Eerden, 1948	Parturition (to hasten delivery): rub body with dried manzanilla and fried onions. Postpartum pains: take as tea. Food: for mother and baby -- take tea.
	<u>M.</u> <u>courrantiana</u> DC.	New Mexico-Spanish	Curtin, 1947	Earache: place warmed, dry flowers in ear with cotton. Neuralgia: apply with warm onion skin. Parturition: take tea to clean out system and for any difficulties. Gonorrhea: take tea. Stomach trouble and fever: take tea
	<u>Matricaria</u> sp.? or <u>Anthemis</u> sp.?	New Mexico-Spanish	Shulman and Smith, 1962	Heartburn: take tea. Colic: take tea to prevent as well as a cure. Stomachaches: take tea.
	<u>Matricaria</u> sp.	New Mexico-Spanish	Ford, 1966	Stomachache: take as tea (3). Colds: take as tea (3). Food: give sweetened tea to babies (3). Suppositories: see Azufre.

	<u>Anthemis</u> sp.	Arizona	Kearney and Peebles, 1964	
	<u>Matricaria</u> sp.	Chihuahua-Juarez	Jones, 1932	Stomach tonic: make infusion
	<u>Matricaria</u> sp.	Chihuahua-Juarez	Ford and Ford, 1965	Infants: boil in water to make tea for babies (8)
	<u>Matricaria matricariodes</u> (Less.) Porter	Baja California-Paipai	Owen, 1963	Frío: drink tea; boil and inhale fumes; and/or use to massage. Menstrual difficulties: take tea.
	<u>Malvaviscus</u> sp.	Durango-Durango	Riley and Trujillo, 1956	Kidney troubles and cloudy urine: see Aceitilla for recipe
(also called Manzanita)	<u>Arctostaphylos pungens</u>	Chihuahua-Tarahumar	Pennington, 1963b	Food: eat fruit. Bronchitis or other pulmonary infection: make tea from leaves.
	<u>Arctostaphylos pungens</u>	Chihuahua-Tepehuán	Pennington, 1963a	Food: drink tea made from leaves as stimulant. Colds: take tea.
	unidentified	San Luís Potosí-Charcas	Whiting, 1934	Food: boil and take
	unidentified	Coahuila-Saltillo	Lundell, 1934	Colic

Spanish Name	Botanical Name	Location	Reference	Use
	unidentified	Durango-Llano Grande near La Ferreria	Riley and Trujillo, 1956	Tuberculosis: boil tops, stems, and leaves until water is tinted; sweeten and take 3 times a day for 8 days
450. Manzanilla Bollona	unidentified	Chihuahua-Tepehuán	Pennington, 1963a	Diarrhea: take tea made from leaves
451. Manzanilla del Campo	*Zinnia pumila* Gray	San Luís Potosí-Charcas	Whiting, 1934	
452. Manzanilla de Castilla	*Matricaria courrantiana* DC.	Chihuahua-Chihuahua	Zingg, 1932	Douche: women use hot decoction
453. Manzanilla del Río	*Gnaphalium Wrightii*	Chihuahua-Tarahumar	Pennington, 1963b	Diarrhea: take tea made from leaves and flowers. Cough: same as above.
	Gnaphalium Wrightii Gray	Chihuahua-Chihuahua	Zingg, 1932	Colds: take decoction. Sores and ulcers: use decoction as wash.
	Gnaphalium sp.	Chihuahua-Tarahumar	Bennett and Zingg, 1935	
	Gnaphalium sp.	Chihuahua-Tepehuán	Pennington, 1963a	Stomach disorders: take decoction of leaves. Dysentery: take decoction of leaves.

	G. Maccounii	Chihuahua-Tepehuán	Pennington, 1963a	Heart pains and coughing: see Gordolobo
454. Manzanita	Ribes inebriens Lindl.	New Mexico-Cochiti	Lange, 1959	Food: eat berries
	Ribes inebriens Lindl.	New Mexico-Tewa	Robbins, et al., 1916	Food: eat fruit
	Arctostyphylos uva-ursi (L.) Spreng.	New Mexico-Spanish	Curtin, 1947	Venereal disease, rheumatism, anemia, stomach trouble: see Coralillo.
	A. pungens	Chihuahua-Tarahumar	Pennington, 1963b	Food: see Manzanilla. Bronchitis: see Manzanilla.
	A. pungens	Baja California-Paipai	Owen, 1963	Stomachache and vomiting: drink tea made from root
455. Maravilla	Quamoclidion multiflorum Torr.	New Mexico-Spanish	Curtin, 1947	Goitre: use ground root. Sore throat: blow powdered root into throat or take hot bath. Fever: mix powdered leaves with white vaseline and rub over whole body. Mumps: crush roots and apply mixed with lard. Rheumatism: apply powdered roots on affected areas with

Spanish Name	Botanical Name	Location	Reference	Use
				camphorated oil. Dropsy: grind roots and rub on body or drink decoction with Punche, Poñil, and cornmeal.
(Raiz de Maravilla)	Mirabilis multiflora (Torr.) Gray	New Mexico-Spanish	Ford, 1966	Rheumatism: grind root into powder and rub on affected areas (3)
456. Margarita	Karwinskia humboltiana Zucc.	Western Mexico	Rose, 1899	Fever: crush leaves, soak in water, drink cold infusion
457. Marihuana	Cannabis sativa L.	New Mexico-Spanish	Curtin, 1947	Rheumatism: grind leaves and rub on body as counter-irritant
(Marijuana)	Cannabis sativa L.	Baja California-Paipai	Owen, 1963	Colic
458. Mariola	Artemisia rhizomata A. Nels.	New Mexico-Spanish	Curtin, 1947	Pregnancy and to expell afterbirth: take powdered leaves with water. Stomach pains: chew fresh or dry leaf or make tea.
	Artemisia sp. [sagebrush]	New Mexico-Spanish	Shulman and Smith, 1962	Throat ailment. Constipation: use as laxative.

	Parthenium incanum H.B.K.	Arizona	Kearney and Peebles, 1964	
	Parthenium incanum H.B.K.	San Luís Potosí-Charcas	Lundell, 1934	Stomach trouble: use as bitters
	Parthenium incanum H.B.K.	Nueva Leon-Monterrey	Lundell, 1934	
	unidentified	Chihuahua-Parral	Riley and Trujillo, 1956	Rheumatism: boil in water and take; grind and mix with hot oil and apply. Disinfectant for water: place herb in water (10 gm/5-10 liters water for 8 days).
459. Mariquilla	*Solidago canadensis* L.	New Mexico-Spanish	Curtin, 1947	Sore throat: mash fresh plant and mix with soap and bind to throat
460. Marrubio	*Marrubium vulgare* L.	New Mexico-Spanish	Curtin, 1947	Chilblains, frozen feet and rheumatism: boil leaves to make hot foot bath. Sores: apply dry, powdered leaves alone or with lard. Stomachache and colic: add starch to tea and take as mush. Coughs: make syrup by adding sugar and honey to tea. Fever and pneumonia: take syrup?

Spanish Name	Botanical Name	Location	Reference	Use
	Marrubium vulgare L.	San Luís Potosí-Charcas	Whiting, 1934	Rheumatism. Sleep. Fright: place under mattress.
	Marrubium vulgare L.	Nueva Leon-Monterrey	Lundell, 1934	
	Marrubium vulgare L.	Western Mexico	Rose, 1899	Rheumatism: make liniment from leaves and add mescal
	Marrubium vulgare L.	Valley of Mexico-Tepepan	Madsen, 1965	Stomachache: for recipe see Cedrón
461. Masarquite (Hoja de Lantén)	unidentified	Durango-La Ferreria	Riley and Trujillo, 1956	Dysentery: boil until water tinted, take each a.m. for 9 days or until cured. (Can mix with Lengua de Vaca and Yerba de Pajaro)
462. Mastránzo	_Marrubium vulgare_ L.	New Mexico-Spanish	Curtin, 1947	see Marrubio
	Marrubium vulgare L.	New Mexico-Spanish	Ford, 1966	Infections (external) and boils: boil and apply (3)
(Mastránso)	_Marrubium vulgare_ L.? [horehound]	New Mexico-Spanish	Shulman and Smith, 1962	Throat ailments. Infections. Sore throat: blow smoke in patient's throat.

463. Mata	*Eupatorium arizonicum* A. Gray	New Mexico-Spanish	Curtin, 1947	Smoking: add leaves to tobacco -- supposedly intoxicating
464. Mata Guasano	*Cosmos Pringlei*	Chihuahua-Tarahumar	Pennington, 1963b	see Bavisa
465. Matarique	*Cacalia decomposita* Gray	Chihuahua-Tarahumar	Bennett and Zingg, 1935	Diabetes. Colds: pound plant, boil for tea. Wounds: use decoction as wash. Purgative: grind roots and drink with warm water. Fish poison.
	Cacalia decomposita Gray	Chihuahua-Chihuahua	Zingg, 1932	Diabetes
	Cacalia sp. (Mano de Leon)	Zacatecas-Zacatecas	Riley and Trujillo, 1956	Kidney trouble, veneral disease, diabetes: boil roots and take each morning for 9 days
466. Matariqui	*Cacalia decomposita*	Chihuahua-Tarahumar	Pennington, 1963b	Rheumatism: boil crushed roots, strain, drink liquid. Wounds: use crushed roots in poultice. Caries: place piece of root in cavity. Malaria and other fever: take tea made from roots and leaves.

Spanish Name	Botanical Name	Location	Reference	Use
	unidentified	Chihuahua-Juarez	Jones, 1932	Kidney disorders: boil roots and use liquid
467. Mate (see Yerba Mate)				
468. Mejorana	*Origanum* sp.?	New Mexico-Spanish	Ford, 1966	Food: use as seasoning herb (1)
	Origanum sp.?	Chihuahua-Juarez	Ford and Ford, 1965	Food: use in cooking (8)
	unidentified	San Luís Potosí-Charcas	Lundell, 1934	Constipation: To give appetite
469. Melon-cilla	*Sida hederacea* (Dougl.) Torr.	New Mexico-Spanish	Wooton and Standley, 1915	
(Melon-silla)	*Sida hederacea* (Dougl.) Torr.	New Mexico-Spanish	Wooton, 1894	
470. Mambrillo, Semilla de	unidentified	Chihuahua-Parral	Riley and Trujillo, 1956	Stomach troubles (children): boil in water and take 3 times a day for 8-9 days
471. Menta	*Menta arvensis*	New Mexico-Spanish	Ford, 1966	
472. Mescal	*Agave* sp.	Baja California-Paipai	Owen, 1963	Menstrual difficulties: toast leaves, make tea; drink each morning of

				period
473. Mesquite	*Prosopis juliflora* var. *torreyana* L. Benson	Baja California-Paipai	Owen, 1963	Inflamed eyes: boil leaves for eyewash; may add salt. Smallpox and measles: boil bark for tea; both purge and emetic. Diuretic.
	P. chilensis (Mol.) Stuntz	San Luís Potosí-Charcas	Whiting, 1934	
(Mezquite, Corteza de)	*P. chilensis* (Mol.) Stuntz	Chihuahua-Chihuahua	Zingg, 1932	Purgative: drink decoction made from bark. Urine: drink decoction of bark to clarify
474. Mezquite Extranjero	*Parkinsonia aculeata* L.	Coahuilla-Torreón	Kelly, 1965	No utility
475. Mezquite Gum	*Prosopis* sp.	Chihuahua-Parral	Riley and Trujillo, 1956	Bad stomach: for recipe see Lenasa, Semillas de
476. Miel	not a plant -- honey	New Mexico-Spanish	Shulman and Smith, 1962	Tonic: use with vinegar for spring tonic
477. Mirasol	*Helianthus annuus* L.	New Mexico-Spanish	Wooton, 1894	
	Helianthus annuus L.	Chihuahua-Tarahumar	Pennington, 1963b	Food: eat seeds in cake form; eat leaves crushed in a mush

Spanish Name	Botanical Name	Location	Reference	Use
	Viguieria heli-anthoides	Chihuahua-Tarahumar	Pennington, 1963b	Food: eat young leaves raw; older leaves boiled
478. Mirto	*Salvia chamaedryoide* Cav.	San Luís Potosí-Charcas	Whiting, 1934	Piles: boil in water
	S. microphylla H.B.K.	Valley of Mex-ico-Tepotzlan	Redfield, 1928	Los aires: for recipe see Alta Reina
479. Mirto del Campo	unidentified	San Luís Potosí-Charcas	Whiting and Lundell, 1934	Biliousness: boil in water and take
480. Mirto de Castilla	*Salvia* sp.	Nueva Leon-Monterrey	Lundell, 1934	Colic
481. Misto	unidentified	San Luís Potosí-Charcas	Whiting, 1934	Bilis (Anger)
482. Misto del Campo	unidentified	San Luís Potosí-Charcas	Whiting, 1934	Bilis (Anger)
483. Molenillo (see Flor de Molenillo)				
484. Monasillo	*Malvaviscus* sp.	Nueva Leon-Monterrey	Lundell, 1934	Cough: use with other herbs
485. Montezuma	unidentified	San Luís Potosí-Charcas	Lundell, 1934	Rheumatism
486. Mora	*Clorophora* sp.	Zacatecas-Zacatecas	Riley and Trujillo, 1956	To stimulate milk pro-duction in nursing

				mothers: boil bark and take before eating for several days. Open sores: boil bark and use liquid as a wash.
487. Moradilla	Verbena ambrosiaefolia Rydb.	New Mexico-Spanish	Curtin, 1947	Back pains: apply powdered plant and pitch. Nerves or rheumatism: drink and bathe in tea made from leaves. Leprosy: apply dry, ground leaves.
	V. wrightii	Chihuahua-Tarahumar	Bennett and Zingg, 1935	Fever: drink decoction of whole plant (except roots)
	Funastrum heterophyllum (Engelm.) Standl.	San Luís Potosí-Charcas	Lundell, 1934	Fever: boil and use to bathe children
	unidentified	Chihuahua-Tepehuán	Pennington, 1963a	Pain with stomach disorders: crush flowers in water and eat
488. Moronel	Lonicera subspicata var. Johnstonii Keck	Baja California-Paipai	Owen, 1963	Bruises and wounds: boil bundle of leaves; when water is red, cool and bathe wounds

Spanish Name	Botanical Name	Location	Reference	Use
489. Mostacilla	*Lepidium alyssoides* A. Gray	New Mexico-Spanish	Curtin, 1947	Wounds on animals: mash plant, mix with powdered lime, and place in wounds to kill worms
490. Mostaza	*Brassica campestris* L.	New Mexico-Spanish	Curtin, 1947	Rheumatism: use to prepare bath. Cold beginning in ribs or shoulder of left side: bind with plaster of ground mustard, flour and water
	Brassica campestris L.	New Mexico-Spanish	Ford, 1966	Stomachache: place seeds in cold water and drink (3). Witches (to keep them away): place seeds with crossed needles in doorway (3)
	Brassica campestris L.	Chihuahua-Tepehuán	Pennington, 1963a	Fever: take tea made from seeds
491. Muérdago	*Struthanthus diversifolius*	Chihuahua-Tepehuán	Pennington, 1963a	Parturition (difficulties): take tea made from leaves
492. Muerto (Añil de Muerto,				

see Flor de Muerto)				
493. Muicle	*Jacobinia spicigera* (Schl.) Bailey	Valley of Mexico-Tepotzlan	Redfield, 1928	Pregnancy: boil in water and take with sugar during pregnancy
494. Mula (de la Mula)	*Eupatorium subintegrum* (Greene)	San Luís Potosí-Charcas	Lundell, 1934 Lundell, 1934	Rheumatism. Medicinal.
495. Musgo	[moss]	New Mexico-Spanish	Curtin, 1947	Sores (supposedly leprosy): rub on sores
496. Nacahuila (see Flor de Nacahuila)				
497. Nacahuite (see Flor de Nacahuite)				
498. Naranjo, Azahar de (flowers) (see Azahar and Flor de Naranja)	*Citris* sp.			
499. Naranjo, Hojas de (leaves)	*Citris* sp.	New Mexico-Spanish	Ford, 1966	

Spanish Name	Botanical Name	Location	Reference	Use
500. Nebada	Nepeta sp.	New Mexico-Spanish	Ford, 1966	Cats: "catnip" (4)
501. Nebrina	Juniperus sp.	New Mexico-Spanish	Ford, 1966 (name)	(4)
			Curtin, 1947 (uses)	Venereal disease, blood purification, and stomach trouble: see Bellota de Sabina (Juniperus sp.)
502. Negrito	Asplenium monanthes L.	Chihuahua-Tepehuán	Pennington, 1963a	Parturition and rheumatic pains: see Calaguala
503. Nogal	Juglans sp.	New Mexico-Spanish	Curtin, 1947	Rheumatism and leg pains: use bark to make decoction for bathing
	Juglans sp.	Chihuahua-Juarez	Jones, 1932	Blood tonic: take infusion of boiled leaves
	Juglans major (Torr.) Heller	Chihuahua-Chihuahua	Zingg, 1932	Food: make beverage from leaves, a tea with sugar
	Acer Negundo L. Negundo interius [box elder]	New Mexico-Tewa	Robbins, et al., 1916	No food or medicinal uses given
504. Nogal de Castilla, Corteza de	Juglans sp.	Zacatecas-Zacatecas	Riley and Trujillo, 1956	Blood tonic: boil bark, add sugar and alcohol and take after meals for 9 days

505. Nopal	_Opuntia_ sp.	New Mexico-Spanish	Curtin, 1947	Food: eat fried lobes or fruit. Swollen neck glands: apply poultice of this, _Datura_ seeds and linseed. Mumps, soreness, congested breasts: remove spines from joints, roast and bind to neck; or split open and apply warm.
	Opuntia sp.	Chihuahua-Tarahumar	Bennett and Zingg, 1935	Food: eat stem and fruits. Abdominal pains: cut off stems, open peel and cross-hatch with knife; sprinkle ground Culantro seeds over and roast by covering with ashes. Put in palm leaf and wrap around waist.
	Opuntia sp.	Baja California-Paipai	Owen, 1963	Broken bones: toast, remove spines from "leaf", slice in half and place half in each side of the fracture. Wounds: apply sliced "leaf" to festering wound or embedded thorn.
506. Nuez	_Juglans_ sp.	New Mexico	Tidestrom and Kittell, 1941	

Spanish Name	Botanical Name	Location	Reference	Use
(Nuez Entera Moscada) or Nuez	*Myristica* sp. [nutmeg]	New Mexico-Spanish	Ford, 1966	Stomach ailments: add to coffee and take (5). Headache: grind and place on top of head (3). Paralysis (one side of face): plaster with film of honey, punche, cinnamon, and nutmeg; also put on cotton and place in ear (3).
(Nueces)	nuts, e.g. *Juglans* sp.	New Mexico-Spanish	Shulman and Smith, 1962	Aire: see Albacar recipe. Susto: see Canela for recipe.
507. Ocalito	*Eucalyptus* sp.	Zacatecas-Zacatecas	Riley and Trujillo, 1956	Asthma: boil and steep leaves in water; sip as needed
508. Ocote	*Pinus* sp.	New Mexico-Spanish	Curtin, 1947	Cough: make syrup by boiling wood in water and adding sugar. Tuberculosis: boil wood until liquid is thick and drink each morning.
	Pinus sp. [pitch]	New Mexico-Spanish	Shulman and Smith, 1962	Venereal disease: boil bark with Yerba de la Golondrina and brown sugar for tea and to bathe sore genital areas. Rheumatic

				pains and cramps: see Hediondilla for recipe.
509. Ocotillo	*Fouquieria fasciculata*	Chihuahua-Tarahumar	Bennett and Zingg, 1935	Washing: make soap from pounded bark
	Fouquieria fasciculata?	Chihuahua-Tepehuán	Pennington, 1963a	Aching gums: use seeds to prepare poultice. Throat disorders: eat flowers.
	Fouquieria fasciculata?	Coahuilla-Torreón	Kelly, 1965	Delayed menstruation: make tea from blossoms. Kidney disorders: same as above.
	unidentified	Chihuahua-Tarahumar	Pennington, 1963b	Espanto (fright): soak scrapings and rub on children to cure
510. Oja de Aurelia (see Yerba de la Golondrina)				
511. Ojasé (see also Hojansen)	*Flourensia cernua* D C.	San Luís Potosí-Charcas	Lundell, 1934	
	unidentified	Zacatecas-Zacatecas	Riley and Trujillo, 1956	Stomachache from over-eating: boil stems and leaves and take as needed

Spanish Name	Botanical Name	Location	Reference	Use
512. Ojo de Aguila	unidentified	Durango-Rincon Grande de Magayal (3 km from La Ferreria)	Riley and Trujillo, 1956	Bruises: boil branches and leaves and apply hot, wet leaves as poultice .
513. Ojo de Chanate	_Rhynchosia pyramidalis_	Chihuahua-Tepehuán	Pennington, 1963a	Pain from internal injuries (from fall): crush black and white seeds, add water and drink. Inflammations: crush and moisten seeds and roots and apply as poultice
514. Ojo de Gallo	_Sanvitalia procumbens_	Valley of Mexico-Tepotzlan	Field, 1953	Venereal disease: boil 3-4 hours and drink 3 times a day before meals. Mix with Pescadito del Cerro (_Selaginella_?).
515. Ojo de Venado	_Mucuna_ sp.	Valley of Mexico-Tepotzlan	Redfield, 1928	Evil eye: use seeds as charms to protect versus evil eye and evil spirits
516. Orégano (or Orégano de la Sierra)	_Monarda menthaefolia_ Graham	New Mexico-Spanish	Curtin, 1947	Food: use leaves for flavoring stews. Coughs: boil and drink hot tea as needed .
	Monarda menthaefolia Graham	New Mexico-San Ildefonso	Curtin, 1947	Headache: rub dry, ground plant on head .

			Fever: rub dry, ground plant over body.
Monarda menthaefolia Graham	New Mexico-Santa Clara	Curtin, 1947	Fever: rub dry, ground plant over body. Sore throat: take decoction of leaves.
Monarda menthaefolia Graham	New Mexico-Spanish	Ford, 1966	Food: use leaves for seasoning. Cough: boil in water and drink as tea (3).
Monarda sp.? [horsemint]	New Mexico-Spanish	Shulman and Smith, 1962	Sore throat: grind with flour and apply to throat. Cough: use as tea. Blood: use as tea to enrich. Food: use to flavor lentils, peas, and meat.
Lippia Berlandieri L. Palmeri	Chihuahua-Tarahumar	Pennington, 1963b	Food: add leaves to mush; boil leaves and eat with beans; add for seasoning
L. Berlandieri	Chihuahua-Chihuahua	Zingg, 1932	Food: pulverize dry leaves and use for seasoning. Colds: drink decoction.
L. Palmeri L. Berlandieri?	Chihuahua-Tarahumar	Bennett and Zingg, 1935	Food: seasoning

Spanish Name	Botanical Name	Location	Reference	Use
517. Orégano del Campo	*Monarda pectinata* Nutt.	New Mexico-Spanish	Curtin, 1947	Food: seasoning. Stomachache.
518. Orégano Mexicano	unidentified	New Mexico-Spanish	White, 1941	
519. Oreja del Gato	*Lathyrus vernus*	Chihuahua-Tepehuán	Pennington, 1963a	Wounds, infections: crush and apply as poultice
	Hieracium Fendleri	Chihuahua-Tepehuán	Pennington, 1963a	Same as above
	unidentified	Chihuahua-Tepehuán	Pennington, 1963a	Wounds and inflammations: use leaves to prepare poultice
520. Oreja del Ratón	*Hieracium Fendleri*	Chihuahua-Tarahumar	Pennington, 1963b	Sores and wounds: bruise fresh or dry leaves and use as poultice
521. Orejuela del Ratón	*Dichondra argentea* Willd.	Chihuahua-Chihuahua	Zingg, 1932	Jaundice: drink decoction. "Frights": drink decoction.
	Euphorbia albomarginate? Torr. and Gray	Coahuilla-Torreón	Kelly, 1965	Stomachache: take with other items in a decoction. Bilis: use with other items to make a fermented beverage.

	<u>Dichondra</u> <u>argentea</u> Willd.	San Luís Potosí-Charcas	Lundell, 1934	Appetite (to increase)
	<u>Dichondra</u> <u>argentea</u> Willd.	Nueva Leon-Monterrey	Lundell, 1934	
522. Oro Volador	gold leaf -- not a plant	New Mexico-Spanish	Ford, 1966	Heart trouble: mix with deer's blood and wine and drink periodically (4)
523. Ortiquilla	<u>Urtica</u> <u>gracilis</u>	Chihuahua-Tarahumar	Pennington, 1963b	Food: eat tiny fresh leaves, raw or boiled
	<u>Tragia</u> <u>nepetaefolia</u>	Chihuahua-Tepehuán	Pennington, 1963a	Fever: prepare lotion and apply to body
	<u>Tragia</u> <u>nepetaefolia</u>	Coahuilla-Torreón	Kelly, 1965	Delayed menstruation: take as tea
524. Ovozuz (see also Palo Amargo)				
525. Oshá	<u>Ligusticum</u> <u>Porteri</u> Coult. and Rose	New Mexico-Spanish	Van der Eerden, 1948	Stomach disorders: use root
	<u>Ligusticum</u> <u>Porteri</u> Coult. and Rose	New Mexico-Spanish	Curtin, 1947	Food: use leaves to season soups. Snake repellent: carry root in pocket and sprinkle powder around bedroll. Snakebite: make paste with root and water;

Spanish Name	Botanical Name	Location	Reference	Use
				apply to draw out poison. Cuts, sores, bruises: use in mixture for ointment. Constipation: use with other items to make suppositories. Colic (children): make tea of leaves. Stomach gas: chew root. Stomachache: grind root, take with water, or make tea. Colds, chronic cough, flu, pneumonia, tuberculosis: take powdered root with hot water, sugar, and whiskey; or syrup from stems. Fever: take tea made from root. Headache: place masticated root on forehead. Enema: use with other ingredients.
	Ligusticum Porteri Coult and Rose? [Indian root]	New Mexico-Spanish	Shulman and Smith, 1962	Infection: carry piece of root to avoid. Rattlesnakes: carry piece of root to ward off. Witch: carry piece of root to ward off. Aire: carry piece of root to protect from cold and aire. Emetic: mix with salt. Stomach trouble.

				Tuberculosis. Broken bones: make paste with wild tobacco (Punche) Rheumatic pains: see Hediondilla. Cramps. Infection of wounds: grind into powder, put on wound to protect.
	Ligusticum _Porteri_ Coult. and Rose	New Mexico-Spanish	Ford, 1966	Cuts: grind root and apply powder (3). Stomach ailments: chew root (3). Suppositories: see Azufre. Snake repellent: carry root (3).
(Chuchupate)	_Ligusticum_ _Porteri_ Coult. and Rose	Chihuahua-Juarez	Ford and Ford, 1965	
526. Otate	Family: _Gramineae_ Tribe: _Bambuseae_	Tamaulipas-Tula	Lundell, 1934	Internal tumors
	Family: _Gramineae_ Tribe: _Bambuseae_	Nueva Leon-Monterrey	Lundell, 1934	Inflammation
527. Otatillo	_Muhlenbergia_ _dumosa_	Chihuahua-Tepehuán	Pennington, 1963a	Stomach cramps: use roots to make tea
528. Pachona	unidentified	Durango-Llano Grande near La Ferreria	Riley and Trujillo, 1956	Scratches, wounds, sores: apply fresh leaves with butter to sore area

Spanish Name	Botanical Name	Location	Reference	Use
529. Pagué	<u>Dyssodia</u> <u>papposa</u> (Vent.) Hitchc.	New Mexico-Spanish	Curtin, 1947	Indigestion, diarrhea, vomiting: steep leaves to make tea. Stomachache: chew leaves. Colic (babies): soak seeds in hot water and give to drink.
	<u>Pectis</u> sp.? <u>Dyssodia</u> <u>papposa</u> [fetid marigold]	New Mexico-Spanish	Shulman and Smith, 1962	Stomachache. Diarrhea.
	<u>Dyssodia</u> <u>papposa</u> (Vent.) Hitchc.	New Mexico-Spanish	Ford, 1966	Diarrhea: boil flowers in water and drink (3). Stomachache: take as tea (1).
530. Palma	<u>Yucca</u> sp.	New Mexico-Spanish	Curtin, 1947	See Amole
	<u>Yucca</u> <u>decipiens</u>	Chihuahua-Tarahumar	Pennington, 1963b	Food: use roots and leaves to make cheese. Washing: use roots for soap.
(Sotol)	<u>Dasylirion</u> <u>durangense</u>	Chihuahua-Tarahumar	Pennington, 1963b	Food: toast and eat stems; also use to make tesguino
(Sotol)	<u>D</u>. <u>Wheeleri</u>	Chihuahua-Tarahumar	Pennington, 1963b	Food: as above. Headache: roll scrapings from emerging flower-

				stalk into small balls and apply
	Sabal uresana	Chihuahua-Tarahumar	Pennington, 1963b	Food: eat heart raw or roasted
Palma, Flor de (see Flor de Palma)				
531. Palma Chino (see Flor de Chino)				
532. Palma de San Pedro	*Yucca decipiens*	Chihuahua-Tepehuán	Pennington, 1963a	Purgative: mash seeds and take them with warm water
533. Palmilla	*Yucca* sp.	New Mexico-Spanish	Curtin, 1947	see Amole
	Yucca decipiens	Chihuahua-Tarahumar	Pennington, 1963b	see Palma
	Yucca elata	New Mexico-Spanish	Wooton and Standley, 1915	Washing: use root for soap
	Yucca elata	New Mexico-Spanish	Kearney and Peebles, 1964	Food: eat young flower stalks and lower stem
	Dasylirion durangense	Chihuahua-Tarahumar	Pennington, 1963b	see Palma

Spanish Name	Botanical Name	Location	Reference	Use
	D. Wheeleri	Chihuahua-Tarahumar	Pennington, 1963b	see Palma
	Nolina durangensis	Chihuahua-Tarahumar	Pennington, 1963b	Fiber and glue: no food or medicinal uses given.
	N. matapensis	Chihuahua-Tarahumar	Pennington, 1963b	same as above.
	N. durangensis	Chihuahua-Tarahumar	Bennett and Zingg, 1935	Baskets
534. Palmilla Ancha	Yucca sp.	New Mexico-Spanish	Curtin, 1947	see Amole
	Y. baccata	New Mexico-Tewa	Robbins, et al, 1916	see Amole
535. Palms	Palmaceae	New Mexico-Spanish	Shulman and Smith	Palms blessed on Palm Sunday; burn, drink ashes mixed with water.
536. Palo Amargo (Palo Orozuz)	unidentified	New Mexico-Spanish	Ford, 1966	
537. Palo Amarillo	Berberis fremontii Torr.	New Mexico-Spanish	Curtin, 1947	Tuberculosis: boil roots and add to bath. Rheumatism and pains in ribs: boil broken branches, drink and bathe in liquid.

				Jaundice: same as for rheumatism. Fevers: "cold plant" so good for fever. Charm vs. lightning: wear cross of the wood on chest and back.
	Tecoma stans	Chihuahua-Tarahumar	Pennington, 1963b	Colds: decoct flowers into a tea. Heart pains: employ as a rubbing compound on chest.
538. Pala Anacahuite	_Cordia_ sp.	Zacatecas-Zacatecas	Riley and Trujillo, 1956	Bronchial troubles: boil wood and take liquid 3 times/day for 3-4 days
539. Palo Apestoso	_Karwinskia humboltiana_	Chihuahua-Tarahumar	Pennington, 1963b	Food: see Cacachila. Fever: see Cacachila.
540. Palo Azul	_Eysenhardtia polystachya_	Nueva Leon-Monterrey	Lundell, 1934	Medicinal wood
541. Palo Babosa	unidentified	Chihuahua-Tepehuán	Pennington, 1963a	Fever: crush roots and add to water and take.
542. Palo Blanco	_Encelia farinosa_ Gray	SW U.S.A.	Beal, 1943	See Incienso
	Celtis sp.	New Mexico	Tidestrom and Kittell, 1941	
	Sapindus	Zacatecas-Zacatecas	Riley and Trujillo, 1956	Upset stomach: boil in water and take twice daily for

Spanish Name	Botanical Name	Location	Reference	Use
				3-4 days.
543. Palo Brazil (see Brazíl)				
544. Palo Cenizo	Buddleia tomentella	Chihuahua-Tepehuán	Pennington, 1963a	Diarrhea: use leaves to make tea
545. Palo Colorado	Caesalpinia platyloba	Chihuahua-Tarahumar	Pennington, 1963b	No uses given for food or medicine
546. Palo de Diablo	Bocconia arborea	Chihuahua-Tepehuán	Pennington, 1963a	Sores, wounds and goitres: moisten leaves; crush and use as poultice. Headache: apply crushed leaves to forehead. Stomach upsets: use scrapings of the bark to make a tea. Styes: use scrapings as poultice.
547. Palo Duro	Cercocarpus montanus Raf.	New Mexico-Spanish	Curtin, 1947	Bedbug repellent: keep leafy twigs around beds or insert in mattress in little bags. Paint: use root for paint and tinting hides.
	Cercocarpus montanus Raf.	New Mexico-Tewa	Robbins, et al, 1916	Laxative: mix leaves or whole young plant with salt and powder by pounding; stir

				in cold water and drink.
	<u>Cercocarpus montanus</u> Raf.	Chihuahua-Tarahumar	Pennington, 1963b	Colds, constipation, dysentery: take tea made from leaves. Sores: make poultice from ground roots.
	<u>Celtis reticulata</u> Torr.	New Mexico-Tewa	Robbins, et al, 1916	Food: eat berries
548. Palo Mulato	<u>Bursera grandifolia</u>	Chihuahua-Tarahumar	Bennett and Zingg, 1935	Dysentery: boil bark to make decoction
	unidentified	New Mexico-Spanish	White, 1941	
549. Palo de Ocote	<u>Pinus</u> sp.	New Mexico-Spanish	Curtin, 1947	Tuberculosis and cough: see Ocote
550. Palo Orozuz (Palo Amargo)	unidentified	New Mexico-Spanish	Ford, 1966	
551. Palo Tres Costillas (Lomo de Toro)	<u>Serjania triquetra</u>	Zacatecas-Zacatecas	Riley and Trujillo,1956	Kidney inflammation: soak in water overnight; drink before breakfast each morning for 9 days
552. Paloma Consulta	<u>Thalictrum fendleri</u>	Chihuahua-Tepehuán	Pennington, 1963a	Stomach cramps: boil leaves and stems; take as tea. Fever: take tea of leaves

Spanish Name	Botanical Name	Location	Reference	Use
				and stems or make lotion to bathe.
553. Pamita	_Descurainia pinnata_ ssp. _menziesii_	Baja California-Paipai	Owen, 1963	Indigestion (empacho). Stomachache and vomiting. Children: mix raw seeds with cooking oil and give to children to collect "the bad like mercury collects gold."
554. Papa Cimarron	_Solanum jamesii_ Torrey	New Mexico-Spanish	Curtin, 1947	Food: eat tubers
555. Papache	_Randia echinocarpa_	Chihuahua-Tarahumar	Pennington, 1963b	Food: eat fruits; use bark as tesquino catalyst
	Randia echinocarpa	Chihuahua-Tarahumar	Bennett and Zingg, 1935	Food: eat fruit; bark same as above
556. Papache Grande	_Randia watsonii_	Chihuahua-Tarahumar	Pennington, 1963b	Food: same as Papache--see above
557. Papas	_Solanum tuberosum_ L.	New Mexico-Spanish	Curtin, 1947	Headache: apply slices of raw potato to forehead
	Solanum tuberosum L.	New Mexico-Spanish	Shulman and Smith, 1962	Fever: apply raw slices to forehead
	Solanum tuberosum L.	New Mexico-Spanish	Ford, 1966	Headache: apply raw slices to forehead

558. Paraca	*Cassia skinneri*	Valley of Mexico-Tepotzlan	Field, 1953	Kidney diseases, difficult micturition, blood in urine: boil plant in 2 liters of water 3 times/day before meals, mix with rasposa
559. Parraleña	*Dyssodia setifolia* (Lag.) Robinson	San Luís Potosí-Charcas	Whiting, 1934 Lundell, 1934	Stomachache, constipation, cough; in water
	Dyssodia sp.	Zacatecas-Zacatecas	Riley & Trujillo, 1956	Constipation and coughs: boil branches & flowers & take before meals for 2-3 days.
560. Paschtle	*Tillandsia recurvata* L.	San Luís Potosí-Charcas	Whiting, 1934	
561. Pasmo (see also Yerba del Pasmo)	*Baccharis* sp.	Chihuahua-Tarahumar	Bennett and Zingg	Coughs and colds: take decoction of stems and leaves. Wounds and sores: apply hot poultice to reduce swelling.
	unidentified	New Mexico-Spanish	White, 1941	
	unidentified	San Luís Potosí-Charcas	Lundell, 1934	Chills and gas pains: fry in grease and apply to bowel region

Spanish Name	Botanical Name	Location	Reference	Use
562. Pastora (Yerba de la Vaca, Yerba del Vercerro)	unidentified	Zacatecas-Zacatecas	Riley and Trujillo, 1956	Stomachache: boil stems and flowers and take 3 times/day for 9 days
563. Pata de Callo	*Capriola dactylon*	Durango-El Torreón (near La Ferreria)	Riley and Trujillo, 1956	Headaches: smear fresh leaf with mentholated salve and place on temple; or crumble dry leaf into salve, place on paper and apply to temple.
564. Pata de Leon	*Geranium mexicanum*	Valley of Mexico-Tepepan	Madsen, 1965	"Chincual" (hot illness of babies): treat with cool herbs-make tea with this, and Yerba Mora; give as drink and use to bathe.
565. Pata de Ves Res?	*Cassia bauhinioides* Gray	San Luís Potosí-Charcas	Whiting, 1934 Lundell, 1934	Laxative: -- mild for small children. Stomachache: boil in water and take.
566. Patita de León	*Geranium atropurpurem* Heller	New Mexico-Spanish	Curtin, 1947	Teeth: chew roots to preserve teeth
567. Patito del Campo or (Patito	*Lathyrus decaphyllus* Pursh	New Mexico-Spanish	Curtin, 1947	Toothache, mumps, headache: grind fruit, add dry ground Contrayerba (Kallstroemia).

del País)				and spread on face to reduce swelling and relieve pain. Tonsilitis: grind fruit with Habas, add sugar and blow into throat.
568. Patitos	Acacia greggii A. Gray	New Mexico-Spanish	Curtin, 1947	See Uña de Gato
569. Pato de Gallo	unidentified	Chihuahua-Tarahumar	Pennington, 1963b	Insect bites: use crushed leaves to prepare poultice
570. Paz (see Flor de la Paz)				
571. Pazote	Chenopodium ambrosioides L. var. anthelminticum (L.) Aellen	New Mexico-Spanish	Van Der Eerden, 1948	To increase mother's milk supply
	Chenopodium ambrosioides sp.	New Mexico-Spanish	Shulman and Smith, 1962	Heart: use to prevent heart trouble. Menstrual cramps: use as tea. Aire: use for headaches and dizziness.
(Ipazote)	C. ambrosioides	New Mexico-Spanish	Ford, 1966	Stomachache: chew dry leaves. Food: use to season beans.

Spanish Name	Botanical Name	Location	Reference	Use
	C. ambrosioides	New Mexico-Spanish	White, 1941	
(Pazote Comer)	_Chenopodium_ sp.	Chihuahua-Juarez	Ford & Ford, 1965	Food: cook with beans
(Pazote de Comer)	_Chenopodium_ sp. L.	San Luís Potosí-Charcas	Whiting, 1934	Pain: boil in water
Epazote de Comer; Hipazote	_Chenopodium ambrosioides_ sp. L.	New Mexico-Spanish	Curtin, 1947	Emmenagogue: use leaves to make suppositories. To abort, relieve pains after childbirth and to regulate catamenial distress: chew leaves with salt and swallow. To produce milk, make blood flow, to relieve post-partum pains: take as tea. Blood purification: drink decoction. Appendicitis: use rectal suppositories with several other ingredients. Food: use seeds to season meats.
(Epazote)	_Chenopodium ambrosiodies_ sp. L.	Valley of Mexico-Tepepan	Madsen, 1965	Anger sickness: (in uncomplicated cases) treat with purge made with this and magnesium.

Ipasote	*Chenopodium* sp.	Durango-Durango	Riley and Trujillo, 1956	Coughs and Asthma: take tea made from flowers and stems early in the morning.
	Chenopodium sp.	Durango-Llano Grande near La Ferreria	Riley and Trujillo, 1956	Dysentery: boil leaves with water, add sugar and chocolate; drink as needed.
(Ipazote)	*Chenopodium ambrosioides*	Chihuahua-Tarahumar	Pennington, 1963b	Fever: make decoction from leaves. Stomachache: same as above. Worms: give strong doses of tea to children and animals.
	Chenopodium ambrosioides var.	Chihuahua-Tepehuán	Pennington, 1963a	Parturition (to facilitate): use leaves to make tea. Intestinal worms: take tea.
	unidentified	Baja California-Paipai	Owen, 1963	Stomachache: drink tea
(Ipazote de Comer)	unidentified	Nueva Leon-Monterrey	Lundell, 1934	Medicinal herb
(Ipazote Sarrillo)	*Chenopodium* sp.	San Luís Potosí-California	Lundell, 1934	Chills (after getting wet): boil and drink
(Pazotede Sorillo)	unidentified	Chihuahua-Juarez	Ford and Ford, 1965	Tea
(Ipazote del Zorillo)	*Chenopodium incisum* (L.) Poir.	West Mexico	Rose, 1899	Colic: take as tea. Pneumonia: take as tea.

Spanish Name	Botanical Name	Location	Reference	Use
	Chenopodium incisum (L.) Poir.	New Mexico	Tidestrom and Kittell, 1941	
572. Pazotillo	Erigeron canadensis L.	New Mexico-Spanish	Curtin, 1947	Cosmetic (for clear, white complexion): mash and soak leaves; rinse face with strained liquid; dry; apply coat of powder
573. Pegapega (also called Buena Mujer)	Mentzelia multiflora A. Gray	New Mexico-Spanish	Curtin, 1947	Rheumatism: grind and rub on limbs. Back pains: pulverize and make poultice with water.
(also called Yerba del Buey)	Grindelia aphanactis Rydb.	New Mexico-Spanish	Curtin, 1947	Rheumatism: crush and apply fresh plants. Kidney disorders: boil buds or flowers and take with sugar. "Cold in the bones": place hot water on dry twigs and apply with hot adobe as steamy poultice to aches. Paralysis: use for hot bath Cold: take tea. Stomach trouble: take as tea.
	Mentzelia hispida Willd.	San Luís Potosí-Charcas	Whiting, 1934	Urinary trouble: take in powdered form

574. Peistón	Coleosanthus sp.	Durango-Durango	Riley and Trujillo,1956	Overeating: bring to boil, drink each morning and afternoon for 3 or 9 days
575. Peña, Flor de (see Flor de Peña)	unidentified	New Mexico-Spanish	White, 1941	
576. Peonia	Zexmenia podocephala	Chihuahua-Tarahumar	Pennington, 1963b	Stomach upsets: decoct root into mixture and take. Fish poison.
	Zexmenia podocephala	Chihuahua-Tepehuán	Pennington, 1963a	Purgative: crush roots and add to warm water
	Lantana involucrata	Chihuahua-Tarahumar	Bennett and Zingg, 1935	? Disease that eats in from outside: mix ground roots with lard and use as ointment. Compacted stomach: pound and cook roots to make a drink. Parturition: pound roots and cook to make decoction taken during childbirth. (Mexicans farther south boil leaves with barley and give to women.)
	Peonia sp.	Valley of Mexico-Tepotzlan	Redfield, 1928	Restlessness during fevers: for recipe see Flor de Nacahuite

Spanish Name	Botanical Name	Location	Reference	Use
Piania	_Perezia_ _rancinatalas_	San Luís Potosí-Charcas	Lundell, 1934	Chest troubles: boil and mix with other herbs
577. Perejil	_Petroselinum_ _crispum_ (parsley)	New Mexico-Spanish	Ford, 1966	
	unidentified	Nùeva Leon-Monterrey	Lundell, 1934	Heart
578. Pericón	_Tagetes_ _florida_ Sweet	Valley of Mexico-Tepotzlán	Redfield, 1928	Bathing: steep flowers in water and use to wash new-born babies. Also, new mother may use for bathing.
	Tagetes _florida_ Sweet	Valley of Mexico-Tepotzlan	Field, 1953	Bathing: as above. Colic: boil 2-3 hours, add alcohol and take 3 times/day before meals or give by spoonful to babies.
579. Perula	unidentified pepper tree--_Schinus?_	Baja California-Paipai	Owen, 1963	Swollen members. Frío: make tea and either drink, use for massage, or inhale fumes. ?
580. Pescaditos del Cerro	_Selaginella_ ? _cuspida_	Valley of Mexico-Tepotzlan	Field, 1953	Venereal disease: for re-cipe see Ojo de Gallo
581. Pescado, Raiz de	unidentified	New Mexico-Spanish	Ford, 1966	

582. Peston	*Brickellia* sp.	Chihuahua-Chihuahua	Zingg, 1932	Purgative: boil and take decoction
	Eupatorium sp.	San Luís Potosí-Charcas	Whiting, 1934	Stomach trouble: take powdered in water
	Eupatorium sp.	San Luís Potosí-Charcas	Lundell, 1934	Constipation
583. Pétales de Yolozochitl (Flor de Corazon)	*Talauma mexicana*	Zacatecas-Zacatecas (from Oaxaca)	Riley and Trujillo, 1956	Heart attack and palpitations: boil petals and take 3 times/day for several days
584. Peyote	*Lophophora williamsii*	Chihuahua-Tarahumar	Hrdlička, 1908	Fractures. Open wounds: Snakebite. Orchitis: chew and apply.
	Lophophora williamsii	Chihuahua-Tarahumar	Pennington, 1963b	Bruises, bites, wounds: chew green plants and apply. Rheumatic pains: mix juice with water, drink and use for rubbing.
	Lophophora williamsii	Coahuila-Torreón	Kelly,1965	Sorcery: powder and use to cause mental upset. Shoulder pains. Vaginal discharge.
585. Peyote cimarrón	*Ariocarpus fissuratus*	Chihuahua-Tarahumar	Pennington, 1963b	Bruises, bites, wounds: chew plant and apply
586. Picaro	*Bidens* sp.	San Luís Potosí-	Whiting, 1934	

Spanish Name	Botanical Name	Location	Reference	Use
		Charcas		
587. Pichichagua	Perezia nana Gray	San Luís Potosí-Charcas	Lundell, 1934	Urinary system ? Rat poison: boil in water.
588. Pico Pajaro	Lycium schaffneri Gray	San Luís Potosí-Charcas	Whiting, 1934	
589. Pico de Pajaro	Rhus microphylla Engelm.	San Luís Potosí-Charcas	Whiting, 1934	
590. Piedra, Flor de (See Flor De Piedra)				
591. Piedralipe (Piedra Azul)	not a plant-copper sulphate	New Mexico-Spanish	Ford, 1966	Treat wheat and corn seed before planting
592. Piloncillo	from Saccharum officinarum [crude brown sugar]	New Mexico-Spanish	Shulman and Smith, 1962	Sweetener: often added to teas
593. Pimienta (Pimienta Entera)	?Piper nigrum L. [black pepper]	New Mexico-Spanish	Van Der Eerden 1948	Parturition (to hasten delivery of baby): take internally.
	Piper nigrum L.	New Mexico-Spanish	Ford, 1966	Food: use for seasoning. Coughs: take with warm water.

				Stomachache: take with warm water
594. Pinavete	*Pinus ponderosa* Lawson, var. *scopulorum* Engelm. *P. brachyptera* Engelm.	New Mexico-Tewa	Robbins, et al, 1916	
595. Pinguay	*Hymenoxys richardsonii* (Hook.) *Cockerell* var. *floribunda* (Gray) K.F. Parker *H. floribunda* (A.Gray)	New Mexico-Cochiti	Lange, 1959	Gum: chew bark and/or roots
(Pingué or Pinhué)	*Hymenoxys floribunda* A. Gray	New Mexico-Spanish	Curtin, 1947	Gum: peel roots and chew inner pulp
	Hymenoxys richardsonii (Hook.) Cockerell var. *floribunda* (Gray) K.F. Parker	New Mexico-Spanish	Shulman and Smith, 1962	Unspecified remedy
	H. floribunda (A. Gray)	New Mexico-Spanish	Ford, 1966	Gum: chew roots
596. Pino Macho	*Juniperus sibirica*	New Mexico-Spanish	Curtin, 1947	Fever, thin blood, stomach-ache, colic: see Sabino Macho
597. Pino Real	*Pseudotsuga taxifolia* (Poir.) Britton *P. mucronata*	New Mexico-Tewa	Robbins, et al, 1916	No food or medicinal uses given

Spanish Name	Botanical Name	Location	Reference	Use
598. Pino Real Colorado	*Pinus brachyptera* Engelm.	New Mexico-Spanish	Curtin, 1947	Smallpox pustules and Scaly skin: rub on fresh sap. Liver spots on face: apply oil from small resin blisters with a small brush. Food: use inner bark for food during famine (Indians). Tanning: use bark.
599. Piñon (see also Trementina de Piñon)	*Pinus edulis* Engelm.	New Mexico-Spanish	Curtin, 1947	Syphilis: boil needles in water, add Pilloncillo, place outside overnight, drink 1 glass 3 times/day. Food: toast and eat nuts. Fuel: use wood.
600. Pionilla (Pionillo)	unidentified	New Mexico-Spanish	Ford, 1966	
	unidentified	Baja California-Paipai	Owen, 1963	Stomachache and vomiting: take tea made with a crushed piece of root & hot water
601. Pirul	*Schinus molle* L.	Nueva Leon-Monterrey	Lundell, 1934	Medicinal herb
	Schinus sp.	Durango-El Torreón (near La Ferreria)	Riley and Trujillo, 1956	Backache: grind leaves, mix with warm cooking oil and apply as hot poultice

602. Pirun	Schinus molle L.	Valley of Mexico-Tepotzlan	Redfield, 1928	Rheumatism: steep leaves in water and apply to affected parts of body
603. Pita	Agave sp.	Coahuila-Torreon	Kelly, 1965	Fiber
604. Pitahaya Barbón (also called Pitahaya Viejo)	Cephalocereus leucocephalus	Chihuahua-Tarahumar	Pennington, 1963b	Food: eat fruits and also use to make tesguino
605. Pitajaya	Opuntia imbricata (Haw.) DC.	New Mexico-Spanish	Curtin, 1947	See Entraña (another name for same species)
	Echinocereus paucispinus	New Mexico-Spanish	Curtin, 1947	Swelling and Dropsy: boil blossoms and take 3 times/day
	Lemaireocereus	Chihuahua-Tarahumar	Bennett and Zingg, 1935	Food
606. Plumahilla	Achillea lanulosa Nutt.	New Mexico-Cochiti	Lange, 1959	Chills: put leaves in cold water for a day to make tea; drink until cured
(Plumajillo)	Achillea lanulosa Nutt.	New Mexico-Spanish	Curtin, 1947	Fever ("cold" plant so good for fever): mix dry leaves with Lantén (Plantago) leaves; grind, put in

Spanish Name	Botanical Name	Location	Reference	Use
				boiling water and drink. Purge: if drink too much tea.
				Cough: swallow dry flowers with water twice each day. Sprains and broken bones: make poultice from whole plant.
	<u>Achillea</u> <u>lanulosa</u> Nutt. [yarrow]	New Mexico-Spanish	Shulman and Smith, 1962	Stomache. Fever: use as tea Dizziness: with Poléo, use as tea and as solution for bathing. Constipation: use as laxa-tive.
	<u>Achillea</u> <u>lanulosa</u> Nutt.	New Mexico-Spanish	Ford, 1966	Stomach ailments: make tea and drink
	<u>Achillea</u> <u>lanulosa</u> Nutt.	California-Spanish	Curtin, 1947	Cuts and bruises: steep leaves in water and apply. To stop flow of blood: use as in previous item.
607. Pochote	<u>Ceiba</u> <u>acuminata</u>	Chihuahua-Tarahumar	Pennington, 1963b	Food: toast seeds and add to atole gruels, eat roots and and drink liquid from roots

608. Polellito Chino	Hedeoma oblongifolia	New Mexico-Spanish	Ford, 1966	
609. Poléo	Mentha sp.	New Mexico-Spanish	Curtin, 1947	Fever: mash with vinegar and salt and spread over body. Miscarriage: eat leaves after miscarriage.
	Hedeoma nanam Torr.	New Mexico-Spanish	Ford, 1966	Fever: make tea and drink
	Mentha sp.	California-Spanish	Curtin, 1947	Excessive menses: mix with sage. Catarrh (chronic): toast and grind leaves and stems with inmortal, rosilla seed pods; mix with suet and rub salve on forehead, nose, neck. Also, snuff up nose a tea of leaves and inmortal leaves, stems, and roots.
	unidentified [mint pennyroyal]	New Mexico-Spanish	Shulman and Smith, 1962	Fever: mix with soda and vaseline and rub on. Dizziness: see Plumajillo for recipe. Aire, headaches, and dizziness.
	Mentha canadensis	Chihuahua-	Pennington,	Stomach pains: use crushed

Spanish Name	Botanical Name	Location	Reference	Use
		Tepehuán	1963a	leaves to make tea
	Cunila longiflora ?	Chihuahua-Juarez	Jones, 1932	Food: make a beverage for babies
	unidentified	Chihuahua-Juarez	Ford and Ford 1965	Insomnia: take as sedative
	unidentified	Chihuahua-Tepehuán	Pennington, 1963a	Catarro (influenza): take as tea
610. Poléo Chino	Hedeoma oblongifolia (Gray) Heller	New Mexico-Spanish	Curtin, 1947	Emmenagogue: take decoction of whole plant. Fever: ("cold" plant so good for fever) mix powdered dry leaves with cold water and drink daily. Stomach trouble: chew green plant. Teeth: chew green plant.
611. Poléo Chinito	unidentified [mint pennyroyal]	New Mexico-Spanish	Shulman and Smith, 1962	See Poléo
612. Poléo Grande (Poléo de: País)	Mentha canadensis L.	New Mexico-Spanish	Curtin, 1947	Food: use leaves for flavor-ing. Fever: steep leaves and give liquid to children to drink and/or rub dry, ground leaves with vaseline on body. Fever with neck pains: rub

				on dry leaves and inmortal. Colds: apply poultice of ground leaves and hot water on back of neck or chest. Stomachache: take tea.
613. Poléo del Monte	unidentified	Chihuahua-Tepehuán	Pennington, 1963a	Coughing spells: take tea
614. Polvitas del Navájo	unidentified	New Mexico-Spanish	Shulman and Smith, 1962	Toothache: apply to bad tooth Stuffed nasal passage: make powder and sniff.
615. Ponso	<u>Tanacetum</u> <u>vulgare</u> L.	New Mexico-Spanish	Curtin, 1947	Cramps, Stomachache: chew leaves or make tea. Chills and fever. Torpid liver: drink decoction.
	<u>Tanacetum</u> sp. [Tansy]	New Mexico-Spanish	Shulman and Smith, 1962	Stomach upset: use as tea
616. Poñil	<u>Fallugia</u> <u>paradoxa</u> [Don] Endl.	New Mexico-Spanish	Curtin, 1947	Cough: boil roots, add sugar and take before meals, in morning and at night. Swelling: use blossoms to make paste with flour, water and Mastránso for massage. Rheumatic joints: rub pulverized leaves mixed with Punche. Hair rinse: boil roots and use as rinse to prevent hair from falling out.

Spanish Name	Botanical Name	Location	Reference	Use
				Versus curse: grind plumes with soot, Sange de Venado, rock salt, add to wine and drink.
	Fallugia paradoxa [Don] Endl.	New Mexico-Tewa	Robbins, et al, 1916	Hairwash: steep leaves and use on hair
617. Popote	Baccharis sp.	Valley of Mexico-Tepotzlan	Redfield, 1928	Toothache: steep roots in alcohol and place on gums
(also called Popotón)	Stipa vaseyi Scribn.	New Mexico-Spanish	Curtin, 1947	Kidney trouble: boil roots and drink tea. Anti-witch charm: use with other items.
618. Popotilla	Ephedra sp.	Zacatecas-Zacatecas	Riley and Trujillo, 1956	Venereal disease, chest diseases, coughs and bronchial ailments: boil branches in water and take hot liquid every 3 hours for 3 days
619. Popotillo	Ephedra torreyana S. Wats.	New Mexico-Spanish	Curtin, 1947	see Cañatilla
	E. antisyphilitica Meyer	Chihuahua-Juarez	Jones, 1932	Stomach medicine: mix infusion of stems with lemon or orange juice and sugar

620.	Popuisoli	Quercus endlichiana	Chihuahua-Tepehuán	Pennington, 1963a	Mouthwash: boil bark to prepare lotion to use as mouthwash
621.	Prodigiosa	Calea zacatechichi	Valley of Mexico-Tepotzlan	Redfield, 1928	Biliousness: boil plant and beat with egg and sugar; drink
	(Atanagia Amarga)	Coleosanthus squarrosus	Zacatecas-Zacatecas	Riley and Trujillo, 1956	Diabetes, lack of appetite,and stomachache: boil in water and take twice each day, take as needed, avoiding sugar; eat plenty of greens and soups.
		Coleosanthus sp.	Chihuahua-Parral	Riley and Trujillo, 1956	Stomach ulcers: take infusion of leaves for 9 days (1 cup before breakfast and 2 before evening meal). Kidney troubles: same as above.
622.	Punche	Nicotiana sp.	New Mexico-Spanish	Van Der Eerden, 1948	Navel of newborn: place on navel after stump of umbilical cord has fallen off. Stomach trouble and fever: for recipe see Ajenjibre.
		N. attenuata Torr.	New Mexico-Spanish	Curtin, 1947	Smoking. Kidney trouble: mix pulverized plant with Yerba de Buey juice and tie over affliction. Post-partum pains: sprinkle with Romero on silk cloth

Spanish Name	Botanical Name	Location	Reference	Use
				fold, heat, apply locally. Rheumatic limbs: mix powdered leaves with ground root of Yerba del Peco and rub on. See also, Poñil. Rheumatism: boil in water and use for sponge bath. Chest cold: mix ground leaves with lard; place on piece of linen and bind to chest. Piles: use to make suppositories with raw fat and salt. Ointment made with Yerba del Manso.
	N. rustica	New Mexico-Spanish	Ruxton, 1847	Smoking
	N. rustica ? [wild tobacco]	New Mexico-Spanish	Shulman and Smith, 1962	Broken bones: use with Oshá and Yerba de la Negrita. Rheumatic joints: apply oil, then cover with leaves and warm cloths.
	N. rustica	New Mexico-Spanish	Ford, 1966	Suppositories: see Azufre. Earache: roll leaves together with Ruda to form cigar; light it; blow smoke into ear. Tick in ear: boil, dab on cotton, place in ear; will

				draw tick out.
623. Punchón	Verbascum thapsus L.	New Mexico-Spanish	Curtin, 1947	Smoking. Asthma: smoke and inhale; soak leaves in whiskey and drink.
624. Quassia (see Cuasia)				
625. Quelite	Amaranthus sp.	New Mexico-Cochiti	Lange, 1959	Food: eat as table greens
	Amaranthus sp.	New Mexico-Tewa	Ford, 1966	Food: eat as greens
(also called Calite de Agua)	Amaranthus retroflexus L. A. graecizans A. blitoides Wats.	New Mexico-Tewa	Robbins, et al, 1916	Food: boil and fry; eat as greens
	Chenopodium sp.	New Mexico-Spanish	Ford, 1966	Food: cook with chile, onion, bacon
	Chenopodium sp.	New Mexico-Tewa	Ford, 1966	Food: eat as greens
(Calite)	Chenopodium album	New Mexico-Spanish	Wooton, 1894	
	Chenopodium album	Chihuahua-	Pennington,	Food: eat cooked, in small

Spanish Name	Botanical Name	Location	Reference	Use
		Tarahumar	1963b	amounts or stomach pains will result (if raw).
	_C_. _ambrosioides_	Chihuahua-Tarahumar	Pennington, 1963b	Food: as above. Fever, stomachache, worms: see Ipazote.
	Solanum nigrum	Chihuahua-Tarahumar	Bennett and Zingg, 1935	Food: cut leaves and boil for greens
626. Quelite Morado	_Amaranthus hybridus_ L.	New Mexico	Tidestrom and Kittell, 1941	
	_A_. _paniculatus_ L.	Chihuahua-Chihuahua	Zingg, 1932	Morning sickness: drink decoction
627. Quelites Colorado Yus (Quelites Yus)	_Amaranthus powellii_ S. Wats.	New Mexico-Spanish	Curtin, 1947	Food: eat leaves as greens
628. Quelite Salado	_Chenopodium album_ L.	New Mexico-Spanish	Curtin, 1947	Food: eat leaves as greens
	Suaeda sp.	Arizona-Pimas and others	Kearney and Peebles, 1964	Food: eat young plants as greens; make pinole from seeds
629. Quina	_Cinchona_ sp.	Zacatecas-	Riley and	Blood tonic: drink decoction

(Quina Roja)		Zacatecas	Trujillo, 1956	of boiled bark, sugar, and alcohol. Chills, fever, sore throat and stomach troubles: boil bark and take decoction. Blood poison and skin swelling: boil bark and use as wash.
630. Raiz de China	*Smilax cordifolia*	?Nueva Leon or San Luís Potosí	Lundell, 1934	
631. Raiz del Desierto	*Glycyrrhiza* sp.	New Mexico	Tidestrom and Kittell, 1941	
632. Raiz del Indio	unidentified	New Mexico-Spanish	Ford, 1966	
	Rumex sp.	Chihuahua-Parral	Riley and Trujillo, 1956	Kidney troubles and VD: boil piece of root and drink 3 times daily before meals. Skin infections: use liquid to wash and sprinkle dry, powdered root on area.
633. Raiz de Lobo	*Helenium Hoopesii* Gray	New Mexico-Spanish		See Yerba del Lobo
634. Raiz del Oso (see Yerba del Oso)	unidentified	New Mexico-Spanish	Ford, 1966	

Spanish Name	Botanical Name	Location	Reference	Use
635. Raiz de Pescado	unidentified	New Mexico-Spanish	Ford, 1966	
636. Raiz de Sangre (see Yerba de la Sangre)	unidentified	New Mexico-Spanish	Ford, 1966	
637. Raiz de Valeriana	*Valeriana* sp.	Zacatecas-Zacatecas	Riley and Trujillo, 1956	Nerve trouble: boil small piece of root in cupful of water; drink liquid to produce sleep. Crush root into alcohol and rub on neck.
638. Rama de Sabina	*Juniperus monosperma* *(Engelm.) Sarg.*	New Mexico-Spanish	Curtin, 1947	Parturition: one month before childbirth, take tea made from twigs each morning. Inflammation of stomach: take tea after letting it set outside overnight. Gripes in the intestines: mash twigs and pour hot water over; strain and drink.
639. Ramon	*Parosela canescens*	San Luís Potosí-Charcas	Whiting, 1934	Regulating the stomach
640. Reina de	*Peniocereus* sp.	Arizona-	Kearney and	Food: eat roots

	la Noche		"Indians"	Peebles, 1964	
641.	Remolino	not a plant[pebbles of resin deposited by bees on rocks]	New Mexico-Spanish	Ford, 1966	Heart trouble: for recipe see Alegría
642.	Renerio	unidentified	New Mexico-Spanish	Shulman and Smith, 1962	Witchcraft: use for witch-caused disease
643.	Retama	unidentified	Durango-Durango	Riley and Trujillo, 1956	Kidney trouble and varicose veins: take tea in mid-afternoon for 9 days
644.	Retana (or Retama)	*Tecoma* sp.	Durango-La Ferreria	Riley and Trujillo, 1956	Kidney trouble: boil leaves and flowers in water and take daily before a meal for 9 days
645.	Rocillo	unidentified	Durango-Rinoir Grande de Magayál	Riley and Turjillo, 1956	Upset stomach and fever: boil leaves in water, sweeten and take before retiring for 3 nights
646.	Romerillo	*Artemisia filifolia* Torr.	New Mexico-Spanish	Curtin, 1947	Rheumatism: boil whole bush in water and use as bath. Lacerations (Penitentes):use tea to wash.
		Artemisia sp. [silversage]	New Mexico-Spanish	Shulman and Smith, 1962	Headaches: use in vapor inhalation

Spanish Name	Botanical Name	Location	Reference	Use
	Artemisia filifolia Torr.	New Mexico-Spanish and Tewa	Curtin, 1947 and Robbins, et al, 1916	Indigestion, flatulence and biliousness: chew and swallow with water or drink in hot decoction. Stomach pains: on stomach compress a bundle of the plant after steeping in boiling water and wrapping in a cloth.
	Artemisia sp.	New Mexico-Spanish	Ford, 1966	Stomach ailments: make powder, boil in water and drink. Suppositories: see Azufre.
647. Romero	Rosmarinus officinalis L.	New Mexico-Spanish	Van Der Eerden, 1948	Navel of newborn: place on navel after stump of umbilical cord has fallen off
	Rosmarinus officinalis L.	New Mexico-Spanish	Shulman and Smith, 1962	Female complaints. Aire: use for headaches and dizziness. Parturition: use in steam bath after delivery to restore female fecundity. Penitentes wounds: use in brew to soak whips to avoid bad wounds.
	Rosmarinus officinalis L.	New Mexico-Spanish	Ford, 1966	Colds: boil in water and drink

Rosmarinus officinalis L.	New Mexico-Spanish	Marquez, 1964	Post-partum hemorrhage: use with heated bricks to fumigate
Rosmarinus sp.	Durango-Varal near la Ferreria	Riley and Trujillo, 1956	Nail infections: grind leaves and mix with crebo de riñonada (a commercial salve) and apply to sore area
Trichostema parishii	Baja California-Paipai	Owen, 1963	Bruises and wounds: make salve with Trementina, ground Romero and another herb; use as dressing. Stomachache and vomiting: make tea from the leaves and drink. Empacho: take tea of leaves. Constipation: use as purge. Frio: drink tea; use for massage; and/or boil and inhale fumes. Menstrual difficulties: take tea of leaves.
unidentified	Chihuahua-Juarez	Jones, 1932	Incense: priests use in services
unidentified	Coahuila-Saltillo	Lundell, 1934	Stomachaches
unidentified probably _Rosmarinus_	San Luís Potosí-Charcas	Lundell, 1934	Snake and insect repellent: burn in house to chase out

Spanish Name	Botanical Name	Location	Reference	Use
	Rosmarinus officinalis L.	Chihuahua-Juarez	Ford and Ford 1965	
648. Romero de Castilla	_Chrysanthemum balsamita_ L.	New Mexico-Spanish	Curtin, 1947	Mouthwash: boil with crushed pecan meats and shells. Uterine hemorrhage: boil handful with quart of red wine heat a brick, put in a vessel, and cover with the liquid. Stand patient, wrapped in sheet, over steam until relief is obtained.
649. Romero Cedro	_Cowania_ sp.	New Mexico-Spanish	Tidestrom and Kittell, 1941	
650. Rosa Cimarron (also called Rosa del Campo)	_Rosa fendleri_ Crépin	New Mexico-Spanish	Curtin, 1947	Sore throat: mix ground petals with sugar and blow into throat with paper tube. Skin trouble: (eczema): mix ground petals with wildcat fat and apply. Fever blisters: apply dry powder.
651. Rosa de Castilla	_Rosa_ sp.	New Mexico-Spanish	Curtin, 1947	Sore throat: take powdered red petals with sugar and butter. Swallow dried powdered leaves of the yellow variety. Fever: boil dry or fresh

				yellow petals and take with sugar when cool.
	Rosa sp.	New Mexico-Spanish	Shulman and Smith, 1962	Earaches and broken ear drums: use flower petals.
	Rosa sp.	New Mexico-Spanish	Ford, 1966	Fever: use petals to make tea and drink. Sore throat or fever blister: place petals in mouth.
	Rosa sp.	Nueva Leon-Monterrey	Lundell, 1934	Medicinal herb
	Rosa sp.	Baja California-Paipai	Owen, 1963	Inflamed eyes: boil leaves into a tea and use as eyewash (salt may be added). Stomachache and vomiting: drink tea. Constipation: boil 1 flower in cup of water; drink. Menstrual difficulties: for recipe see Cilantro.
	Rosa centifolia	Valley of Mexico-Tepepan	Madsen, 1965	Empacho: part of complex treatment
652. Rosa de San Pedro	*Macrosiphonia hypoleuca* (Benth.) Muell. Arg.	Chihuahua-Chihuahua	Zingg, 1932	Infected eyes: use decoction to bathe eyes
653. Rosabari	*Artemisia ludovicana*	Chihuahua-	Pennington,	Menstruation: take tea of

Spanish Name	Botanical Name	Location	Reference	Use
		Tarahumar	1963b	leaves during menstrual period
654. Rosatilla (Rositilla)	unidentified	New Mexico-Spanish	Ford, 1966	
655. Roseta	Cenchrus pauciflorus	New Mexico-Spanish	Curtin, 1947	Food: use decoction of whole plant to prepare blue cornmeal mush. Good to increase lactation in nursing mothers.
	C. tribuloides L.	New Mexico-Spanish	Wooton, 1894	
656. Rosetilla	Franseria acanthicarpa (Hook.) Coville	New Mexico-Spanish	Curtin, 1947	(Name used only at Chimayo--see Yerba del Sapo for uses.)
	F. hookeriana Nutt.	New Mexico-Spanish	Wooton, 1894	
657. Rosita	Gutierrezía Sarothrae (Pursh) Britt. & Brown	San Luís Potosí-Charcas	Whiting, 1934	
658. Rosita Morada	Phlox nana	New Mexico-Spanish	Curtin, 1947	Fever blisters: apply ground petals. Dye.

659. Ruda	*Ruta graveolens* L.	New Mexico-Spanish	Curtin, 1947	Deafness: make cigarette with leaves and blow smoke in ear. Nerves and neuralgia: mix with tobacco and smoke as cigarette. Earache: heat leaves and apply with drops of oil. Headache (with cold): smoke as cigarette or place over coals and inhale. Stomach upset: take as tea.
	Ruta sp. [Rue]	New Mexico-Spanish	Shulman and Smith, 1962	Dizziness: smoke . Deafness: use to prevent . Earache: mix (dried) with olive oil, place in ear.
	Ruta sp.	New Mexico-Spanish	Ford, 1966	Earache: roll leaves with Punche to form a cigar; light and blow smoke into ear
	R. graveolens L.	Valley of Mexico-Tepotzlan	Robbins, 1928	Abdominal pains: boil with Mirto (*Salvia*) and Poléo de Monte (?) Los aires: use as a wash.
	R. chalepensis L.	Chihuahua-Mexico City	Zingg, 1932	Air in the intestines and stomach: take decoction
	unidentified	probably San Luís	Lundell, 1934	Headache: to let air out of head

Spanish Name	Botanical Name	Location	Reference	Use
		Potosí-Charcas		
	Ruta sp.	Chihuahua-Juarez	Ford and Ford, 1965	
660. Ruda Cimarron (also called Ruda de la Sierra)	Thalictrum fendleri Engelm.	New Mexico-Spanish	Curtin, 1947	Headache (with cold): smoke as cigarette or sprinkle on coals and inhale; place head on pillow of dry leaves.
661. Sabila	Agave bovicornuta	Chihuahua-Tepehuán	Pennington, 1963a	Sores (from worms) on animals: crush flowers and add to sap from crushed leaves; use as poultice. Toothache: place sap from leaves on cheek and hold there by a rag for a few minutes.
662. Sabina	Juniperus monosperma (Engelm.) Sarg.	New Mexico-Spanish	Curtin, 1947	See Rama de Sabina.
	Juniperus monosperma (Engelm.) Sarg.	New Mexico-Tewa	Robbins, et al 1916	Post-parturition: boil leaves and drink liquid and use to bathe on 3rd day after birth. Tooth decay: use gum to fill cavity.

				Food: eat berries. Diuretic: decoct berries in water. Any Internal chill: berries are "hot" and thus, good for any internal chill.
(Sabino Tree)	Taxodium mucronatum	Zacatecas-Zacatecas	Riley and Trujillo, 1956	Varicose veins: boil seeds and use as wash as well as take cup nightly
663. Sabina Macho	Juniperus sibirica Burgsd.	New Mexico-Spanish	Curtin, 1947	Fever: drink decoction of dry or fresh leaves. Thin blood: same as above. Stomachache and colic: boil small piece of branch to make tea; take hot.
	Juniperus communis L.	New Mexico-Spanish	Shulman and Smith, 1962	Colds: use tea. Blood: use tea for thin blood. Fever: use tea. Colic: use tea.
	Juniperus communis L.	New Mexico-Spanish	Ford and Ford, 1965	Urinary disorders: make tea from needles and drink (3)
	unidentified	Chihuahua-Juarez	Ford and Ford, 1965	
664. Saca Manteca	Solanum madrense	Chihuahua-Tepehuán	Pennington, 1963a	Inflamations: use to prepare poultice

Spanish Name	Botanical Name	Location	Reference	Use
665. Sacahuista	Nolina microcarpa Wats.	Arizona- "Indians"	Kearney and Peebles, 1964	Food: eat caudex and emerging flower stalk
666. Sacate Chino	Hilaria cenchroides H.B.K.	San Luís Potosí-Charcas	Whiting, 1934	
667. Sacate Cochonollo	Cenchrus pauciflorus Benth.	San Luís Potosí-Charcas	Whiting, 1934	
668. Sacate Cola Sorra	Lycurus phleoides H.B.K.	San Luís Potosí-Charcas	Whiting, 1934	
669. Sacate Masarca	Panicum obtusum H.B.K.	San Luís Potosí-Charcas	Whiting, 1934	
670. Sacate Sevaidilla	Sitanion Hystrix (Nutt.) J.G. Smith	San Luís Potosí-Charcas	Whiting, 1934	
671. Sacatón	Stipa vaseyi Scribn.	New Mexico- Spanish	Curtin, 1947	See Popote (Popotón)
	Sporobolus Wrightii Munro	San Luís Potosí-Charcas	Whiting, 1934	
	Sporobolus sp.	Arizona	Kearney and Peebles, 1964	
672. Sagui (Sagu)	unidentified	New Mexico- Spanish	Ford, 1966	
673. Sal	?not a plant [table salt]	New Mexico- Spanish	Shulman and Smith, 1962	Wounds: use on suppurating wounds.

				Fallen fontanelle: use to pack.
674. Salavata	not a plant--soda	New Mexico-Spanish	Shulman and Smith, 1962	Mumps: mix with vinegar and apply paste to neck
675. Salvarial	*Salvia apiana* Jeps.	Baja California-Paipai	Owen, 1963	Stiff neck: tie leaves around neck. Coughs and colds: boil leaf into tea and drink.
676. Salvarial de la Sierra	*Salvia pachyphylla* Epl. ex Munz.	Baja California-Paipai	Owen, 1963	Coughs and colds: boil leaf into tea and drink
677. Salvía	*Buddleia scordiodes* H.B.K.	Coahuila-Torreón	Kelly, 1965	Delayed menses: take in emulsion. Empacho: give tea to babies Bilis: ferment in tequila with other herbs and take.
	? *Salvia hispanica* or *tiliaefolia*	Chihuahua-Parral	Riley and Trujillo, 1956	Stomach troubles: boil and take infusion in morning before eating for 3 days
	unidentified	New Mexico-Spanish	Ford, 1966	
	unidentified	Nueva Leon-Monterrey	Lundell, 1934	Food (babies): boil in water and milk and give
	unidentified	Durango-Rio Grande near La Ferreria	Riley and Trujillo, 1956	Corns: apply fresh leaf to corn and bind; or grind dry leaves and mix with lard to

Spanish Name	Botanical Name	Location	Reference	Use
				make paste (corn will fall off in 3 days)
	unidentified	Durango-Rio Grande near La Ferreria	Riley and Trujillo, 1956	Stomachaches: boil in water; take a cup of liquid each day before breakfast
678. Samán	_Coursetia_ _glandulosa_ Gray	Chihuahua-Tarahumar	Bennett and Zingg, 1935	
679. Samo	_Willardia_ _mexicana_	Chihuahua-Tarahumar	Pennington, 1963b	Dysentery: dry and pulverize the gum on the bark; infuse and drink. Fever: as above.
680. San Diego Florde (See Flor de San Juan)				
681. San Juan (See also Flor de San Juan)				
682. San Nicolás	_Chrysactinia_ _mexicana_ Gray	Coahuila-Torreón	Kelly, 1965	Fertility: take in decoction with other items
	Chrysactinia _mexicana_ Gray	San Luis Potosí-Charcas	Lundell and Whiting, 1934	Chills (in women) from exposure: take as tea
	Chrysactinia _mexicana_ Gray	Nueva Leon-Monterrey	Lundell, 1934	Parturition: (?) for women having children take with

				other herbs
	Menodora coulteri Gray	San Luís Potosí-Charcas	Whiting, 1934	
683. San Rafael	unidentified	San Luís Potosí-Charcas	Lundell, 1934	Sweat bath and to prevent going to sleep after eating
684. Sanaparicio	unidentified	San Luís Potosí-Charcas	Lundell, 1934	Fever
685. Sangre de Cristo (also called Sangre de Drago)	*Berberis repens*	New Mexico-Spanish	Curtin, 1947	See Yerba de Sangre
	Jatropha cardiophylla (Torr.) Muell. Arg.	Arizona "Indians"	Kearney and Peebles, 1964	Bleeding wounds: use clear sap to stop bleeding. Hide tanning: use root - also red dye.
686. Sangre Grado	*Jatropha curcas* L.	West Mexico	Rose, 1899	Purgative: use seeds
686. Sangre de Venado	*Calamus Draco* [Rattan Palm]	New Mexico-Spanish	Curtin, 1947	Paralysis: mix with dried Barbasco, nutmeg, cinnamon; drink some with warm water and use rest to make paste with olive oil to rub on members. Neuralgia or shooting pains:

Spanish Name	Botanical Name	Location	Reference	Use
				mix with ground Azahar, wine and hueso de licor and drink.
	Blood from deer	New Mexico-Spanish	Ford, 1966	Heart trouble: for recipe see Oro Volador. Heart trouble: for other recipe see Alegría.
688. Sangrinaria	Hypericum pratense Schlecht.	Valley of Mexico-Tepotzlan	Redfield, 1928	Costumbre blanca (white menses) in pregnant women: boil with Thryallis glauca and 2 other plants
	Helianthemum glomeratum	Valley of Mexico-Tepotzlan	Field, 1953	Costumbre blanca (white menses) and for men with white discharge: boil, sweeten, add another herb and drink before meals
	unidentified	New Mexico-Spanish	Ford, 1966	
689. Santa María	Aristolochia brevipes	Chihuahua-Tarahumar	Bennett and Zingg, 1935	Fevers: pound root and boil in water
	unidentified	Durango-Rio Grande near La Ferreria	Riley and Trujillo, 1956	Sore throat: boil leaves and stems, sweeten and take hot at breakfast for 5 days
690. Santa Rita (See also Flor de Santa Rita)	unidentified	New Mexico-Spanish	Ford, 1966	

691. Saramago	Brassica Eruca L. Eruca sativa	San Luís Potosí-Charcas	Whiting, 1934	
692. Saranda	Boerhaavia mirabilis	Chihuahua-Tepehuan	Pennington, 1963a	Fever: take strong tea made from leaves
	unidentified	Chihuahua-Tepehuan	Pennington, 1963a	Fever: take weak tea made from leaves
693. Sarza (see Zarza)	Humulus lupulus neo-mexicanus Nels. & Ckll.	New Mexico-Spanish	Curtin, 1947	See Zarza
694. Sasafras	Sassafras sp.	New Mexico-Spanish	Ford, 1966	Blood tonic: drink as tea (1)
695. Sauce	Chilopsis linearis (Cav.) Sw. var.	Coahuila-Torreón	Kelly, 1965	Fever: use decoction as enema
696. Sauco (Flor de Sauco)	Sambucus mexicana Presl	Baja California-Paipai	Owen, 1963	Inflamed eyes: boil in a tea and use as eyewash (salt may be added). Fever and Influenza: boil dry flowers into a tea. Stomachache and vomiting: take as tea.
(Sauca)	Sambucus mexicana Presl	Valley of Mexico-Tepotzlan	Redfield, 1928	Eye trouble: for recipe see Aceitilla
	Sambucus mexicana	Chihuahua-Parral	Riley and Trujillo, 1956	Whooping cough; bronchial troubles: boil seeds, take before eating.

Spanish Name	Botanical Name	Location	Reference	Use
				Body sores: mix crushed seeds with water, boil to make paste; spread on cloth and apply to sore area.
(See also Flor de Sauco)	*Sambucus caerula*	Chihuahua-Tepehuán	Pennington, 1963a	Fever: take tea made from flowers. Heart trouble: take as tea. Cuts or bruises: apply poultice made from crushed young leaves.
697. Saumyate	*Castilleja arvensis* C. and S.	Valley of Mexico-Tepotzlan	Redfield, 1928	Los aires: for recipe see Alta Reina
698. Sauz, Flor de (See Flor de Sauco)				
699. Savila	*Aloe* sp.	West Mexico	Rose, 1899	Venereal Disease: use crushed leaves with oil to make poultice for swellings
700. Sayas	*Amoreuxia palmatifida* Moc. and Sesse ex DC.	Arizona-Pima, Papago, Mexico	Havard, 1895	Food: roast and eat
701. Scoba	*Aster spinosus* Benth.	New Mexico-Spanish	Wooton, 1894	

702. Sebadilla	Swertia radiata (Kellogg) Kuntze	New Mexico-Spanish		See Cebadilla
703. Semilla(s) Higeron (see also Higuera)	Ricinus communis L.	Nueva Leon-Monterrey	Lundell, 1934	Laxative
704. Semilla de Llantén (see also Llantén)	Plantago major L.	Chihuahua-Chihuahua	Zingg, 1932	Dysentery or diarrhea: boil seeds and drink decoction
705. Semillas de Lenása (Tenosa)	unidentified [linseed] ? Linum sp.	Chihuahua-Parral	Riley and Trujillo, 1956	Bad stomach: boil seeds with mezquite gum and take. Body sores: boil and grind seeds, apply plaster. Hair dressing: boil seeds until gummy, apply to keep hair in place.
706. Sempualillo	unidentified	Durango-San Pedro across river from La Ferreria	Riley and Trujillo, 1956	Tired eyes: use fresh stems and leaves, boil in water; when cool, apply drops to eyes.
707. Seniso (see also Cenizo)	unidentified	Chihuahua-Juarez	Jones, 1932	Stomach medicine: take infusion
	Leucophyllum laevigatem Standl.	San Luís Potosí-Chacas	Lundell, 1934	Medicinal herb

Spanish Name	Botanical Name	Location	Reference	Use
708. Sensitiva	<u>Calliandra</u> <u>humilis</u> var. <u>reticulata</u>	Chihuahua-Tarahumar	Pennington, 1963b	Sleeplessness: eat seeds
709. Sevada (see Cebada)	<u>Hordeum</u> <u>vulgare</u> L.	San Luís Potosí-Chacas	Whiting, 1934	
710. Sevollita del Campo (see Cebollita...)	<u>Allium</u> <u>kunthii</u> G.Don <u>Allium</u> <u>scaposum</u> Benth.	San Luís Potosí-Chacas	Whiting, 1934	
711. Siempre Verde	unidentified	Durango-Rio Grande near La Ferreria	Riley and Trujillo, 1956	Blood tonic (to build up): boil leaves and stems, add lemon juice and sugar and take 3-4 times/day for 4 days
712. Siempre-viva	<u>Sedum</u> sp.	New Mexico-Spanish	Curtin, 1947	Earache: heat leaf and place in ear. Corns: crush leaf and bind on. Backache: mash leaves, heat and apply as poultice on back.
	<u>Sedum</u> sp. ?	New Mexico-Spanish	Shulman and Smith, 1962	Earache: steep, pour liquid in ear
713. Socoyol	<u>Oxalis</u> <u>violacea</u> L.	New Mexico-Spanish	Curtin, 1947	See Chocoyle
(Socoyolle)	<u>Oxalis</u> <u>albicans</u> H.B.K.	Chihuahua-Tepehua	Pennington, 1963a	Fever: take tea made from plant

714. Sóli	unidentified	Chihuahua-Tepehuán	Pennington, 1963a	Cold or fever: crush root and sniff
715. Sonorita	Lantana sp.	West Mexico	Rose, 1899	Parturition: boil leaves with barley and give to women in childbirth
716. Sotol	Yucca decipiens	Chihuahua-Tarahumar	Pennington, 1963b	See Palma
	Dasylirion durangense	Chihuahua-Tarahumar	Pennington, 1963b	See Palma
	D. Wheeleri	Chihuahua-Tarahumar	Pennington, 1963b	See Palma
	D. Simplex	Chihuahua-Tarahumar	Bennett and Zingg, 1935	Use fibre
717. Suelda	Buddleia scordioides H.B.K.	Nuevo Leon-Monterrey	Lundell, 1934	Medicinal herb
718. Tabajillo	Hedeoma piperita Benth.	Valley of Mexico-Tepotzlan	Redfield, 1928	Abdominal pains: boil plant with brown sugar and take liquid
719. Tabardillo	Calliandra californica	Baja California-Paipai	Owen, 1963	Stomachache and bloody stools: grind root, boil in water, and drink copiously
	Piqueria trinervia Cav. ?	West Mexico	Rose, 1899	Typhoid fever: crush leaves, make into an infusion and take. Deafness caused by typhiod: use to relieve.

Spanish Name	Botanical Name	Location	Reference	Use
720. Tachachinole	unidentified	Zacatecas-Zacatecas	Riley and Trujillo, 1956	Inflammation of female genitals: boil leaves and stems; use as douche nightly for 9 days
721. Tamarindo	<u>Tamarindus</u> <u>indica</u> L.	Chihuahua-Juarez	Jones, 1932	Food: dissolve beans in water, add sugar, and drink as beverage. Flavoring: use e.g. in ice cream
	<u>Tamarindus</u> <u>indica</u> L.	Mexico	Martinez, 1959	Fever: use in a mixture
722. Tansé	<u>Tanacetum</u> <u>vulgare</u> L.	New Mexico-Spanish	Curtin, 1947	Stomachic and fever: See Ponso
723. Tapacula	unidentified	Valley of Mexico-Tepotzlan	Field, 1953	Diarrhea and dysentery: boil plant and take liquid 3 times/day
724. Tapona	<u>Lepidium</u> <u>virginicum</u> var. <u>pubescens</u> (Greene) C.L. Hitchc.	Baja California-Paipai	Owen, 1963	Empacho: take tea made from leaves
725. Tarumarra ?visvirindy	<u>Asclepias</u> <u>setosa</u> Benth.	Nuevo Leon-Monterrey	Lundell, 1934	
	<u>Asclepias</u> <u>setosa</u> Benth.	San Luís Potosí-Charcas	Lundell, 1934	

726. Tasajilla	Opuntia leptocaulis DC.	New Mexico-Spanish	Wooton and Standley, 1915	
727. Táscate	Juniperus sp.	Chihuahua-Tepehuán	Pennington, 1963a	Sweatbath for sick person: use branches
728. Tatalencho	Selloa glutinosa Spreng.	San Luís Potosí-Charcas	Lundell, 1934	Rheumatism
729. Tavachín	Caesalpinia pulcherrima	Chihuahua-Tarahumar	Pennington, 1963b	Gonorrhea: use roots to make tea
730. Té	Thelesperma megapotamicum (Spreng.) Kuntz T. gracile A. Gray	New Mexico-Tewa	Robbins, et al, 1916	See Cota
	T. trifidum (Poir.) Britton	New Mexico-Tewa	Robbins, et al, 1916	See Cota
	Bidens ferulaefolia ?	Chihuahua-Tepehuán	Pennington, 1963a	Stomach cramps: take tea
	Cymbopogon sp.	Chihuahua-Juarez	Ford and Ford, 1965	Beverage
731. Té de Coral	Bidens aurea (Ait) Sherff	San Luís Potosí-Charcas	Whiting, 1934	Laxative: boil in water and take

Spanish Name	Botanical Name	Location	Reference	Use
732. Té de la Hormiga (see also Yerba de la Hormiga)	<u>Wedeliella</u> <u>glabra</u> (Choisy) Cockerell	San Luís Potosí-Charcas	Lundell, 1934	Kidney and bladder trouble: boil with other herbs
733. Té de la India (Demeana, Menta Silvestre, Yerba Buena Silvestre)	unidentified	Zacatecas-Zacatecas	Riley and Trujillo, 1956	Stomach pains, mentrual cramps, nerve troubles: boil leaves and stems and take
734. Té de Olor	unidentified	San Luís Potosí-Charcas	Lundell, 1934	Purge: boil in water
735. Té de Sena	<u>Cassia</u> sp.	New Mexico-Spanish	Ford, 1966	Laxative: boil and drink
736. Té Silvestre	<u>Thelesperma</u> <u>gracile</u> A. Gray <u>Thelesperma</u> <u>longipes</u> A. Gray	New Mexico-Spanish	Curtin, 1947	See Cota
737. Teconblate	<u>Condalia</u> <u>spathulata</u> A. Gray	New Mexico-Spanish	Curtin, 1947	Cough: drink decoction of small pieces of plant 3 times/day
738. Tejocote	<u>Crataegus</u> <u>mexicana</u>	Valley of Mexico-	Madsen, 1965	Cough caused by cold: use leaves -- for recipe see

		Tepepan		Caña de Castilla
739. Telempalcate	_Chaptalia semanii_ Hemsl.	San Luís Potosí-Charcas	Lundell, 1934	
740. Tepahuaje	_Leucaena_ sp.	West Mexico	Rose, 1899	To harden gums: use bark
741. Tepalcate	unidentified	New Mexico-Spanish	Shulman and Smith, 1962	Sores: grind and place on open sores
742. Tepeguaje	_Lysiloma Watsoni_	Chihuahua-Tarahumar	Pennington, 1963b	Gonorrhea: boil bark, strain, allow to set; take each morning for 3 months
	Lysiloma Watsoni	Chihuahua-Tepehuan	Pennington, 1963a	Sore gums: boil bark to make wash, hold in mouth
743. Tepopote	_Ephedra Torreyana_ S. Wats.	New Mexico-Spanish	Curtin, 1947	See Cañutilla
744. Teposán	_Buddleia sessiflora_	Chihuahua-Tarahumar	Pennington, 1963b	Boils and sores: apply heated leaves
	Buddleia sessiflora	Chihuahua-Tarahumar	Pennington, 1963a	Menstrual pains: take tea made from leaves and bark. Stomach disorders: take tea made from leaves, bark, roots. Wounds: crush and moisten leaves; use as a poultice.
(Tepozan)	_B. americana_	Valley of Mexico-Tepepan	Madsen, 1965	Bath for new mother (whose bones are cold: Agua de Romero = boil in water with

Spanish Name	Botanical Name	Location	Reference	Use
				rosemary, marigold, leaves of Zapote Blanco, and <u>Schinus mole</u>.
745. Tequesquite	not a plant - crude sodium bicarbonate	New Mexico-Spanish	Curtin, 1947	Food: use in baking and with chile (to prevent heartburn). Distended stomach (flatulence): drink in water.
		New Mexico-Spanish	Ford, 1966	Food: use in baking cookies and cakes
(Tesco)	crude sodium bicarbonate	New Mexico-Spanish	Shulman and Smith, 1962	Stomach cramps
746. Tescalama	<u>Ficus petiolaris</u>	Chihuahua-Tarahumar	Pennington, 1963b	Wounds: use milky excrescence from bark as a wash
	<u>Ficus petiolaris</u>	Chihuahua-Tarahumar	Bennett and Zingg, 1935	Pains in the side: place milk from stem on rag and apply as poultice. Food: eat fruit.
	<u>Hura crepitans</u>	Chihuahua-Tepehuán	Pennington, 1963a	Pains from internal injuries or stings: use gum for poultice. Goitres: apply poultice of gum. Purgative: add gum to warm water and drink.

747. Tianguis	*Alternanthera repens*	Chihuahua-Tarahumar	Pennington, 1963b	Stomach disorders: take tea of leaves. Urine retention : take infusion of pulverized root.
	Alternanthera repens	Chihuahua-Tepehuán	Pennington, 1963a	Stomach disorders: take tea of leaves. Fever: take decoction of crushed roots.
748. Tianguis-pepetla	*Alternanthera* sp.	Valley of Mexico-Tepepan	Madsen, 1965	Typhus: when patient thirsty, give juice from ground herb
749. Tierra de Nuestro - Señor de Esquípula	not a plant-sacred dirt	New Mexico-Spanish	Ford, 1966 Shulman and Smith, 1962	Ailments: dirt from the sanctuary at Chimayo, New Mexico--use internally and externally
750. Tilia Flor de (see Flor de Tilia)				
751. Tilia de Trompo Roja	*Tilia* sp.	Zacatecas-Zacatecas	Riley and Trujillo, 1956	Heart palpitations: boil seed pods and take liquid 3 times/day for several days
752. Timbre ? or Timbé	*Acacia filicioides*	San Luís Potosí-Charcas	Whiting, 1934	Food: use to ferment pulque
753. Tobacco Cimarrón	*Verbascum thapsus* L.	New Mexico-Spanish	Curtin, 1947	See Punchón

Spanish Name	Botanical Name	Location	Reference	Use
	Nicotiana tabacum L.	Valley of Mexico-Tepotzlan	Redfield, 1928	Abdominal pains: use infusion to wash abdomen
754. Tobaco Coyote (Taboco Coyote)	_Nicotiana attenuata_ Torr.	Baja California-Paipai	Owen, 1963	Asthma: smoke to treat difficult breathing
755. Tobaco Loco	_N. trigonophylla_ Dunal	San Luís Potosí-Charcas	Whiting, 1934	Not good for smoking
756. Toloache	_Datura meteloides_ DC. _D. stramonium_ L.	New Mexico-Spanish	Curtin, 1947	Asthma: smoke dry leaves. Lice: grind seeds, mix with fat, and use as salve to remove lice. Boils, pimples, swellings: rub on ointment of ground seeds and suet. Piles: apply powdered leaves. Colds and diarrhea: take hot bath containing plant.
	D. meteloides DC.	Chihuahua-Tarahumar	Pennington, 1963b Bennett and Zingg, 1963	Inflammations and sprains: apply poultice of heated leaves. Headache: apply leaves to forehead.
	D. meteloides	Baja California-	Owen, 1963	Wounds: grind root with a little water and apply to

		Paipai		festering wound to eliminate maggots. Venereal disease: toast root, grind, take as tea. Boils: place leaf on festering boil to make it burst and drain.
	D. stramonium L.	Chihuahua-Tepehuán	Pennington, 1963a	Inflammation, apply heated leaves. Headache: apply poultice of leaves to head. Diarrhea: take decoction of leaves.
757. Tolvache	unidentified	Durango-Rio Grande near La Ferreria	Riley and Trujillo, 1956	Sores: apply fresh leaves to help draw out pus
758. Tomate	Physalis neomexicana Rydb.	New Mexico-Tewa	Robbins, et al, 1916	Food: eat fruit
	Physalis sp.	New Mexico-Spanish	Shulman and Smith, 1962	Unspecified "remedy"
759. Tomate del Campo	Physalis neomexicana Rydb.	New Mexico-Tewa	Robbins, et al, 1916	See Tomate
	P. neomexicana Rydb.	New Mexico-Spanish	Curtin, 1947	Tonsil trouble: grind fruit and mix with a pinch of salt; compress on throat

Spanish Name	Botanical Name	Location	Reference	Use
	P. sordida Fern.	San Luís Potosí-Charcas	Whiting, 1934	
760. Tomatilla	Lycium pallidum Miers.	New Mexico-Tewa	Robbins. et al, 1916	
	Lycium sp.	New Mexico-Spanish and "Indian"	Wooton and Standley, 1915	Food: eat fruit
	Physalis sp.	Chihuahua-Tarahumar	Bennett and Zingg, 1935	Food: eat fruit
761. Tomatillo	Lycium pallidum Miers.	New Mexico-Spanish	Curtin, 1947	See Chico
	Solanum elaeagnifolium Cav.	New Mexico-Spanish	Curtin, 1947	See Tomatillo del Campo
762. Tomatillo del Campo	Solanum elaeagnifolium Cav.	New Mexico-Spanish	Curtin, 1947	To curdle milk: use berries. Swollen tonsils: crush green fruits, mix with salt and bind on throat. Tonsilitis, catarrh, head-ache: blow powder from dry, mature (yellow) fruit into throat via paper tube.
763. Tomatito	Solanum elaeagnifolium Cav.	New Mexico-Spanish	Curtin, 1947	See Tomatillo del Campo

	S. nigrum L.	New Mexico-Spanish	Curtin, 1947	Food: eat fruit
764. Tomatito Pelon	Solanum elaeagnifolium Cav.	New Mexico-Spanish	Curtin, 1947	See Tomatillo del Campo
765. Tomillo (Tomilla)	? Thymus sp.	New Mexico-Spanish	Ford, 1966	
	? Thymus sp.	Chihuahua-Juarez	Ford and Ford, 1965	Food: cook with beans (8)
	unidentified	San Luís Potosí-Charcas	Whiting, 1934	Stomach trouble
766. Torito	unidentified	San Luís Potosí-Charcas	Whiting, 1934	Chest trouble: grind seeds and drink in water
767. Tornillo	Strombocarpa pubescens (Benth.) A. Gray	New Mexico-Spanish	Curtin, 1947	Sore eyes: crush leaves and mix with water for eye-wash. Inflamed eyes (of babies in summer) mix crushed green leaves with mother's milk and place in cloth bag, squeeze liquid in eyes. Inflamation of stomach: chew seeds and swallow with water. Bladder trouble: take tea made from leaves 3 times/day.

Spanish Name	Botanical Name	Location	Reference	Use
	?*Prosopis pubescens* Benth. *Strombocarpa pubescens* (Benth.) A. Gray	Arizona-Pimas	Kearney and Peebles, 1964	Wounds: use bark of roots.
768. Toronjil	*Cedronella mexicana* Benth.	New Mexico-Spanish	Ford, 1966	
	Cedronella mexicana Benth.	Chihuahua-Juarez	Ford and Ford, 1965	Heart: (8)
	Cedronella mexicana Benth.	Mexico City	Ford, 1966	Stomach ailments: take as tea (6)
769. Toronjil de China	*Nepeta* sp.	New Mexico	Tidestrom and Kittell, 1941	
770. Torote	*Fouquieria fasiculata* ?	Chihuahua-Tepehuán	Pennington, 1963a	See Ocotillo
771. Trabul	unidentified	New Mexico-Spanish	Ford, 1966	
772. Tranze	unidentified	New Mexico Spanish	Ford, 1966	
773. Trébol	*Melilotus indica*	Chihuahua-Tepehuán	Pennington, 1963a	Fever: use plant to make tea. Headache: apply dampened leaves to head.

	Melilotus indica	Chihuahua-Tarahumar	Pennington, 1963a	Headache: place crushed and dampened leaves on head
	Trifolium sp.	New Mexico	Tidestrom and Kiddell, 1941	
774. Trebol de Olor	unidentified	Zacatecas-Zacatecas	Riley and Trujillo, 1956	Skin infections: dip flowers in water until tinted and use liquid as wash or on cloth for compress. Genital infections (female): grind flowers, mix with strong vinegar or boil with water, use as a douche. Ulcers of the stomach: drink douche preparation.
775. Trementina	_Pinus_ sp. [pine gum]	Baja California-Paipai	Owen, 1963	Bruises and wounds: see Romero for recipe. Headache: use plaster of pine pitch. Coughs and colds: wrap pitch in cloth and place on chest.
776. Trementina de Piñon	_Pinus edulis_ [piñon pitch]	New Mexico-Spanish	Curtin, 1947	Neuralgia: mix pitch with ground seeds of Yerba del Peco (_Actaea_) and plaster in front and behind ear. Rheumatic joints: rub on dry, ground pitch. Splinters and to draw out pus from wounds: make ointment with pitch and

Spanish Name	Botanical Name	Location	Reference	Use
				other ingredients; apply chewed hard gum on wound to heal after splinter is removed. Headache: mix with salt, Punche; spread on paper and place on temples.
	Pinus edulis	New Mexico-Spanish	Shulman and Smith, 1962	Burns: mix with lysol and oil and use. Cuts: as for burns. Rheumatic pains or cramps: see Gobernadora.
777. Tres Costillas	Serjania triquetra	Valley of Mexico-Tepotzlan	Ford, 1953	White menses in women, to clean out urogenital system in pregnant women, and for men with white discharge: boil in water and drink 3 times /day
778. Trigillo Loco	Avena fatua L.	San Luís Potosí-Charcas	Whiting, 1934	
779. Trigo	Triticum aestivum L.	New Mexico-Spanish	Curtin, 1947	Hair rinse: boil roots and wash hair in liquid
780. Tripa del Cerro	unidentified	Valley of Mexico-Tepotzlan	Field, 1953	Kidney trouble: take decoction

781. Tripa de Judas	Parietaria pennsylvanica Muhl.	Valley of Mexico-Tepotzlan	Redfield, 1928	Internal inflammations: boil and eat entire plant. El daño: see Alta Reina for recipe.
	Parietaria pennsylvanica	San Luís Potosí-Charcas	Lundell, 1934	
782. Trompetilla	Bouvardia sp.	New Mexico	Tidestrom and Kittell, 1941	
783. Trompillo	Solanum elaeagnifolium Cav.	New Mexico-Cochiti	Lange, 1959	Snuff: powder dry berries in fingers and use
	S. elaeagnifolium Cav.	New Mexico-Spanish	Wooton, 1894	
	S. elaeagnifolium Cav.	New Mexico	Wooton and Standley, 1915	Food: use berries to curdle milk
	S. elaeagnifolium Cav.	Arizona-Pimas	Kearney and Peebles, 1964	Food: add crushed berries to milk to make cheese
	S. elaeagnifolium Cav.	Chihuahua-Chihuahua	Zingg, 1932	Food: use berries to curdle milk (after boiling) to make cheese
	S. elaeagnifolium Cav.	San Luís Potosí-Charcas	Whiting, 1934	Eye trouble in goats or burros: put seed in eye
	? Cordia sp.	Durango-Llano Grande near	Riley and Trujillo, 1956	Food: use berries to curdle milk to make cheese

Spanish Name	Botanical Name	Location	Reference	Use
		La Ferreria		
784. Tronadora	unidentified	New Mexico-Spanish	Ford, 1966	
785. Tumba Vaqueras	unidentified	Chihuahua-Parral	Riley and Trujillo, 1956	Epilepsy: boil root and take 3 times/day for 9 days
786. Tumbo Vaqueros (Galusá)	Ipomea sp.	Zacatecas-Zacatecas	Riley and Trujillo, 1956	Heart attacks and kidney infections: boil root and take decoction 3 times/day for 9 days
787. Uña de Gato	Acacia greggii A. Gray	New Mexico-Spanish	Curtin, 1947	Food: suck flowers for honey
	Robinia neomexicana A. Gray	New Mexico-Tewa	Robbins, et al, 1916	No food or medicinal uses given
788. Valeriana	unidentified	Chihuahua-Juarez	Ford and Ford, 1965	Headache: apply root with water to head (8)
789. Vara Blanca (also called Yerba de San Pedro)	unidentified	Chihuahua-Tarahumar	Pennington, 1963b	Rheumatic pains: steep leaves and use as wash
790. Vara Dulce	Baccharis glutinosa	Chihuahua-Tarahumar	Pennington, 1963b	See Jarillo del Río
791. Varas de San José (also	Penstemon torreyi Benth.	New Mexico-Spanish	Curtin, 1947	Whooping cough in babies (when they have paroxysms): boil flowers and sweeten

called Varitas de San José)	*P. torreyi* Benth.			to make syrup. Kidney trouble: boil inflorescence, strain and drink liquid. Cold in chest: same as previous item. Excessive Menses: break plant, boil in water; take 3 swallows and bathe lower part of body in the liquid.
	Castilleja sp.	New Mexico-Spanish	Curtin, 1947	See Flor de Santa Rita. This genus is called Varas de San José at Tesuque.
792. Velas de Coyote	*Opuntia imbricata* (Haw.) DC.	New Mexico-Spanish	Curtin, 1947	See Entraña
	O. imbricata (Haw.) DC.	New Mexico	Wooton and Standley, 1915	
793. Venado (also called Lantén)	*Plantago major* L.	San Luís Potosí-Charcas	Whiting, 1934	
	unidentified	Nueva Leon-Monterrey	Lundell, 1934	Fertility: boil in water and drink
794. Venado Oreja	*Asclepias hypoleucus*	Chihuahua-Tepehuán	Pennington, 1963a	Stomach disorders: take tea made from whole plant. Purgative: take strong tea made from leaves.

Spanish Name	Botanical Name	Location	Reference	Use
795. Venodillo (see Flor de Venodillo)				
796. Ventosidad	<u>Nama</u> sp. ?	New Mexico-Spanish	Ford, 1966	
	<u>Nama</u> <u>undulatum</u> H.B.K.	Chihuahua-Chihuahua	Zingg, 1932	Stomach gas: drink decoction
	<u>N</u>. <u>undulatum</u> H.B.K.	San Luís Potosí-Charcas	Whiting, 1934	Cold: smell, inhale
	<u>N</u>. <u>undulatum</u> H.B.K.	San Luis Potosí-Charcas	Lundell, 1934	Gas pains
	<u>N</u>. <u>Hispidum</u> Gray	Nuevo Leon-Mexican	Lundell, 1934	Stomach trouble
	<u>N</u>. <u>palmeri</u> Gray	San Luis Potosí-Charcas	Whiting, 1934	Catarro: smell, inhale
	unidentified	Durango-Durango	Riley and Trujillo, 1956	Stomachache: boil, take each morning for 4 days
797. Vera Blanca	<u>Croton</u> <u>niverus</u> (?)	Chihuahua-Tarahumar	Bennett and Zingg, 1935	Bladder (to stimulate): boil pounded bark in water, add salt, drink

798. Verbena (Berbena)	*Verbena* sp.	New Mexico-Spanish	Ford, 1966	Stomach ailments: take as tea (3)
	Verbena sp.	New Mexico-Spanish	Shulman and Smith, 1962	Stomach pains and nervous stomach
	V. caroliniana	Chihuahua-Tarahumar	Pennington, 1963b	Boils and contusions: moisten and apply as a poultice leaves or crushed roots. Wounds or boils: make tea from red flowers and take to cure boils or use as a wash for wounds.
	V. ciliata	Chihuahua-Tepehuan	Pennington, 1963a	Fever: take weak tea made from leaves
	V. elegans var. *asperata*	Chihuahua-Tepehuan	Pennington, 1963a	See Alfrombrillo
	unidentified	Chihuahua-Juarez	Ford and Ford, 1965	Sores (8)
	unidentified	Durango-Rio Grande near La Ferreria	Riley and Trujillo, 1956	TB: boil stems and leaves and take in a.m. for 9 days
799. Verdolaga	*Portulaca oleracea*	New Mexico-Cochiti	Lange, 1959	Food: eat as greens
	Portulaca oleracea	New Mexico-Spanish	Ford, 1966	Food: eat as greens (3)

Spanish Name	Botanical Name	Location	Reference	Use
800. Vinagre con Miel	not a plant--vinegar and honey	New Mexico-Spanish	Shulman and Smith, 1962	Tonic: use as spring tonic
801. Vinjora	*Zizyphus acuminata*	Chihuahua-Tarahumar	Pennington, 1963b	Food: eat fruit
802. Vinola	*Acacia cymbispina*	Chihuahua-Tarahumar	Pennington, 1963b	Kidney disorders: take decoction of spines
	A. cochilicantha	Chihuahua-Tepehuán	Pennington, 1963a	Chest pains: take tea made from leaves. Difficulty in urinating: same as above.
803. Vinorama	*Acacia Farnesiana*	Chihuahua-Tarahumar	Pennington, 1963b	Kidney disorders: decoct spines. Headache: mix pulverized buttons (flowers) with grease and rub on head. Bruises: use above as poultice.
804. Violeta	*Viola* sp.	Nueva Leon-Monterrey	Lundell, 1934	Cough: boil with other herbs
805. Visnaga	*Ferocactus Wislizeni* (Engelm.) Britt. and Rose	Mexico	Wooton and Standley, 1915	Food: use pulp interior to make candy
806. Visvirinda	*Castela texana*	San Luís Potosí-Charcas	Lundell, 1934	

807. Wame Goberna-dora	Larrea tridentata (DC.) Coville	Chihuahua-	Zingg, 1932	See Gobernadora
808. Wisachito	Hoffmanseggia densi-flora Benth.	San Luís Potosí-Charcas	Whiting, 1934	
809. Wisapole	Xanthium strumarium var. Canadense (Mill.) T. and G.	Baja California-Paipai	Owen, 1963	"Uncertain medical use"
810. Yedra	Rhus toxicodendron	New Mexico-Spanish	Curtin, 1947	
811. Yedra Grande (also called Yedro del Monte)	Echeveria simulus	Chihuahua-Tepehuán	Pennington, 1963a	Catarro (influenza): take tea of leaves
812. Yerba del Aigre	unidentified	Durango-Llano Grande near La Ferreria	Riley and Trujillo, 1956	Earache: roll leaves and place in ear
813. Yerba del Aire	Trixis sp. cf. radialis	Chihuahua-Tepehuán	Pennington, 1963a	Broken bones: use roots to prepare poultice. Earache: place crushed flowers in ear.
814. Yerba de Alonso García	Dalea formosa Torr.	New Mexico-Spanish	Curtin, 1947	Rheumatism: make tea from plant, drink and use for bath.

Spanish Name	Botanical Name	Location	Reference	Use
				Rickets: give to children as noted for rheumatism.
815. Yerba de Angel	*Waltheria americana*	Valley of Mexico-Tepotzlan	Field, 1953	Jaundice and la bilis: boil, sweeten, add *Polypodium aureum* and drink 3 times/day before meals
	Eupatorium collinum	Valley of Mexico-Tepepan	Madson, 1965	Stomachache from custard apples: make tea with other herbs
816. Yerba Anis	*Tagetes lucida* Cav.	Chihuahua-Chihuahua	Zingg, 1932	Colic and wind on stomach: drink decoction, often take with honey
(Yerba Anis)	unidentified	New Mexico-Spanish	White, 1941	
(see also Yerba Nis)				
817. Yerba de Apache	*Castilleja* sp.	New Mexico-Spanish	Curtin, 1947	See Flor de Santa Rita
818. Yerba del Apache	*Erysimum elatum* Nutt.	New Mexico-Spanish	Curtin, 1947	Pneumonia: chew roots, spit on back and rub in. Rheumatic limbs: mix ground roots with whiskey and water and bind on. Sore throat: blow powdered root into throat.

	Erysimum capitatum (Dougl.) Greene ?	New Mexico-Spanish American	Shulman and Smith, 1962	Pain in chest: use as tea. Illness: use as tea when one feels ill.
819. Yerba del Arriero	*Dyssodia acerosa* DC.	Chihuahua-Chihuahua	Zingg, 1932	Purgative: drink decoction
820. Yerba del Aso	Fam. *Umbelliferae*	Chihuahua-Tarahumar	Bennett and Zingg, 1935	Fever: pound root and take bitter decoction. Chest affections: same as above. Food: roast and eat root, when food shortage.
821. Yerba del Buen Dia	*Sida procumbens* Sw.	San Luís Potosí-Charcas	Lundell, 1934	Boils
	Sida procumbens Sw.	Nuevo Leon-Monterrey	Lundell, 1934	Kidney trouble
822. Yerba Buena	*Mentha spicata* L.	New Mexico-Spanish	Van Der Eerden, 1948	Parturition (to hasten delivery): give to mother in powdered form. Post-partum hemorrhage: drink tea or take in powdered form.
	Mentha spicata L.	New Mexico-Spanish	Curtin, 1947	Indigestion: take as tea, e.g. with cinnamon, cloves, nutmeg. Vermifuge: take decoction. Wounds and sores: use tea as wash.

Spanish Name	Botanical Name	Location	Reference	Use
				Diarrhea: take tea. Neuralgia: take tea. Pre-childbirth: take decoction with cinnamon added.
	<u>Mentha</u> <u>spicata</u> L. ? [spearmint]	New Mexico-Spanish	Shulman and Smith, 1962	Panacea: use for "almost anything." Parturition: use as tea before, during, and after delivery to prevent hemorrhage. Colic: use as tea. Menstrual cramps: tea. Stomachache: tea. Kidney and urinary tract ailments: mix with ginger and honey. Beverage: drink. Rash: give tea to infants to bring out rash. Toothache. Solevacion (fright): use with bicarbonate of soda, nuts, Canela, after massage. Diarrhea: burn, hold baby in smoke. Mix with flour. Poison ivy and pimples: mix with Lysol and use to bathe. Colds: tea. Fever: tea.

Mentha spicata L.	New Mexico-Spanish	Ford, 1966	Stomachache: take as tea. (3) Suppositories: see Azufre.
Mentha spicata L.	Chihuahua-Chihuahua	Zingg, 1932	Indigestion: drink decoction
Mentha spicata L.	Coahuila-Coahuila	Kelly, 1965	Nausea (victim of "air"): take tea with cinnamon. "Perplexed air" and/or Alferecía: rub body with fried mint. Hemorrhage (after miscarriage): use in decoction with other herbs. Intestinal worms: take decoction. Empacho: take decoction.
M. canadensis	Chihuahua-Tarahumar	Pennington, 1963b	Intestinal disorders: take as tea
Mentha sp.	Chihuahua-Tarahumar	Bennett and Zingg, 1935	Toothache: use warm decoction to wash mouth. Gums: apply fresh or dry leaves. Food: eat greens.
unidentified	New Mexico-Spanish	Marquez, 1964	Menstrual cramping and diarrhea: see Collálle for recipe.
unidentified	San Luís Potosí-Charcas	Lundell, 1934	Colic: take as tea

Spanish Name	Botanical Name	Location	Reference	Use
	unidentified	Nueva Leon-Monterrey	Lundell, 1934	Digestion: good for children
	unidentified	Baja California-Paipai	Owen, 1963	Stomachache and vomiting: take tea. Earache: grind dry leaves and place in ears as powder; if ears are draining, make tea of plant and wash well.
823. Yerba del Buey (also called Pegapega)	<u>Grindelia aphanactis</u> Rydb.	New Mexico-Spanish	Curtin, 1947	Many uses: See Pegapega
824. Yerba del Burro	<u>Distichlis spicata</u>	New Mexico-Spanish	Curtin, 1947	Gonorrhea: for recipe see Alfilerillo
825. Yerba del Caballo	unidentified ? <u>Senecio</u> sp.	New Mexico-Spanish	Ford, 1966	Rheumatism: make tea for bath; may use with Collálle or alone (3)
	<u>Senecio filifolius</u> Nutt.	New Mexico-Spanish	Curtin, 1947	Sore throat: make tea and gargle. Rheumatism: for recipe see Coronilla (<u>Gaillardia</u>).
826. Yerba de Caballo	unidentified	Durango-Llano Grande near La Ferreria	Riley and Trujillo, 1956	Colic (in children): roast upper half of a fresh plant and place on stomach until

				it dries
827. Yerba Cabezona	Helenium mexicanum H.B.K.	Coahuila-Torreón	Kelly, 1965	Cold: place bud in nostril to cause sneezing and clear head
828. Yerba de la Cachucha	? Coldenia Greggii (Torr.) Gray	Coahuila-Torreón	Kelly, 1965	"Internal infirmity" of men: boil with other plants
829. Yerba del Cáncer	Cuphea aequipetala	Valley of Mexico-Tepotzlan	Field, 1953	Cancer (skin and stomach) and erysipelas (disipela): boil with alcohol, wash sore, apply powder; drink powder in alcohol
	Acalypha phleoides Cav.	West Mexico	Rose, 1899	Sores: crush leaves and flowers into powder and apply. Itch: take as tea.
	A. hederacea Torr.	Nuevo Leon-Monterrey	Lundell, 1934	Medicinal herb
	A. lindheimeri Muell. Arg.	San Luís Potosí-Charcas	Lundell, 1934	Medicinal herb
(Yerba de Cáncer)	unidentified	Durango-Durango	Riley and Trujillo, 1956	Sores and cancer: use hot liquid to swab area
	unidentified	Chihuahua-Parral	Riley and Trujillo, 1956	Skin sores and wounds: boil stems and leaves; drink and use as a wash

Spanish Name	Botanical Name	Location	Reference	Use
Yerba Cáncer	unidentified	New Mexico-Spanish	White, 1941	
Yerba Cáncer	unidentified	Chihuahua-Juarez	Ford and Ford, 1965	
830. Yerba Candelilla	*Pedilaphthus pavanis* (sic)	? Nuevo Leon or San Luís Potosí, probably	Lundell, 1934	
831. Yerba del Catarro	*Hedeoma dentatum*	Chihuahua-Tarahumar	Pennington, 1963b	Colds: crush roots and leaves, and cup over nose and mouth
832. Yerba Ceniza	*Encelia farinosa*	Southwest United States	Beal, 1943	See Incienso
833. Yerba de Chamizo (but see also Chamiso...)	*Atriplex* sp.	New Mexico-Spanish	Ford, 1966	
834. Yerba del Chivatito	*Chenopodium Botrys* L.	New Mexico-Spanish	Curtin, 1947	Cold in the stomach: steep in boiling water and drink liquid. Bed-wetting in children (to stop): soak small branches in cold water until wine-colored. Drink only this liquid.

	Chenopodium Botrys L. ?	New Mexico-Spanish	Shulman and Smith, 1962	"Female complaints": use as tea. Bed-wetting: use tea to cure.
835. Yerba del Chivato	Pericome caudata A. Gray	New Mexico-Spanish	Curtin, 1947	Rheumatism: boil roots to prepare bath; rub dry, ground leaves on limbs
836. Yerba de Chuparrosa	Erodium cicutarium	Chihuahua-Tarahumar	Pennington, 1963b	Sore throat: drink infusion made from entire plant. Cough and stomachache: same as above. Earache: crush leaves, dampen, place in ear.
837. Yerba Colorada	Eriogonum atrorubens	Chihuahua-Tarahumar	Pennington, 1963b	Pulmonary disorders: boil roots and eat. Astringent: use mashed roots. Toothache: use mashed roots.
	Potentilla Thurberi	Chihuahua-Tepehuán	Pennington, 1963a	See Clameria
(Yerba Colorado)	Rumex crispus L.	Baja California-Paipai	Owen, 1963	Colds: use root to make tea
	unidentified	Chihuahua-Juarez	Ford and Ford, 1965	Beverage: tea (8)

Spanish Name	Botanical Name	Location	Reference	Use
838. Yerba de la Congrena	Acalypha california Benth.	Baja California-Paipai	Owen, 1963	Skin eruptions: make tea from leaves; use as a wash on serious lesions, such as "cancer"
839. Yerba del Coyote	Leptodactylon sp.	Chihuahua-Tepehuán	Pennington, 1963a	Fever: use leaves
	Galium sp.	Chihuahua-Tepehuán	Pennington, 1963a	Stomach disorders: use leaves to make tea
	Euphorbia sp.	West Mexico	Rose, 1899	Rheumatic pains: make tea from dried plant
840. Yerba de la Cucaracha	Haplophyton sp.	Arizona	Kearney and Peebles, 1964	Insecticide: mix dried leaves with molasses
841. Yerba Dulce	Lippis dulcis Trev.	Valley of Mexico-Tepotzlan	Redfield, 1928	Coughs: for recipe see Cabellito del Angel
842. Yerba del Empacho	Chorizanthe fimbriata Nutt.	Baja California-Paipai	Owen, 1963	Stomachache and vomiting: boil root as tea. Empacho: boil whole plant, add toasted deer hooves, burned earth, salt; strain and drink. (See also Bachata)
843. Yerba de la Flecha	Sapium biloculare (Wats.) Pax in Engl.	Arizona and Sonora-Apache,	Kearney and Peebles, 1964	Arrow poison: Apaches use. Fish poison: Mexican Indians use.

		Mexican Indians		
	<u>Sapium</u> <u>biloculare</u> (Wats.) Pax in Engl.	Chihuahua-Tarahumar	Pennington, 1963b	Purgative: add milky juice from bark to water and drink. Fish poison.
	<u>Sebastiania</u> <u>Pringlei</u>	Chihuahua-Tarahumar	Pennington, 1963b	Same as previous item
844. Yerba Fría	<u>Sanvitalia</u> <u>aberti</u> A. Gray	New Mexico-Spanish	Curtin, 1947	Stomach trouble: take decoction of leaves. Stained teeth: chew flowers. Note: flower is cold to taste - use as refrigerant.
	[low growing yellow aster]	New Mexico-Spanish	Shulman and Smith, 1962	Constipation: use leaf as laxative
845. Yerba de la Gallina	<u>Helianthemum</u> <u>glomeratum</u>	Chihuahua-Tarahumar	Bennett and Zingg, 1935	Fever: drink decoction
846. Yerba del Gato	<u>Croton</u> <u>corymbulosus</u> Engelm.	San Luís Potosí-Charcas	Whiting, 1934	"Susto" (fright): boil in water
847. Yerba Gobernadora (see Gobernadora)				

Spanish Name	Botanical Name	Location	Reference	Use
849. Yerba de la Golondrina (see also Golondrina)	<u>Euphorbia</u> <u>serpyllifolia</u> Pers.	New Mexico-Spanish	Curtin, 1947	Tonsilitis: placed crushed with a little salt green (or moistened dry) leaves on throat. Rash: apply fresh plant. Sore throat: gargle with decoction of fresh leaves. Rattlesnake bite: use plant as poultice and drink decoction of leaves.
(also called Oja de Aurelia)	<u>Euphorbia</u> sp.	New Mexico-Spanish	Shulman and Smith, 1962	Heart ailments: boil with 1/2 inch of pine bark and brown sugar. Venereal disease: use as tea and for bathing sore genitals.
	<u>Euphorbia</u> sp.	New Mexico-Spanish	White, 1941	
	<u>Euphorbia</u> sp.	Chihuahua-Tarahumar	Pennington, 1963b	Sores, wounds, inflammations, bruises: make infusion of pulverized leaves and use as wash
	<u>Euphorbia</u> sp.	Chihuahua-Chihuahua	Zingg, 1932	Boils and ulcers on skin: use decoction as wash; grind up dry leaves and dust on cleaned lesion

	E. maculata	Chihuahua-Tepepan	Pennington, 1963a	Aching feet, sores, wounds, inflammations: boil plant and use liquid as lotion
	Euphorbia sp.	West Mexico	Rose, 1899	Swellings and sores: boil and use as a poultice
Yerba de la Golon-drina	Euphorbia prostrata	Durango-La Ferreria	Riley and Trujillo, 1956	Body sores: take infusion twice daily before meals for 9 days. Dysentery: take infusion 3 times/day for 9 days before meals.
849. Yerba del Golpe	Oenothera rosea	Chihuahua-Tepepan	Pennington, 1963a	See Amapola
	O. mexicana Spach	Valley of Mexico-Tepotzlan	Redfield, 1928	Bruises: make infusion and use as wash
	Gaura coccinea Nutt.	San Luís Potosí-Charcas	Lundell, 1934	
	Gaura coccinea Pursh	San Luís Potosí-Charcas	Whiting, 1934	Bruises: place leaves over area; also, boil in water and use to bathe
	G. sinuata Nutt.	Nueva Leon-Monterrey	Lundell, 1934	
	Scoparia sp.	Durango-Durango	Riley and Trujillo, 1956	Injuries caused by blows: boil and use to wash

Spanish Name	Botanical Name	Location	Reference	Use
850. Yerba Gordolobo (see Gordolobo)	unidentified	Baja California-Paipai	Owen, 1956	Bruises: make tea (add salt) and drink for internal bruises
851. Yerba del Guaye	*Grindelia* sp. ? [gum weed]	New Mexico-Spanish	Shulman and Smith, 1962	Colds: boil and drink for colds or when one feels a cold coming
852. Yerba Hechicera	unidentified	Baja California-Paipai	Owen, 1963	Stiff neck: tie leaves around neck. Stomachache and vomiting: make tea and drink. Coughs and colds: take tea.
853. Yerba de la Hormega	*Acalypha phleoides* Cav.	San Luís Potosí-Charcas	Whiting, 1934	
	Wedeliella glabra (Choisy) Cockerell	Nueva Leon-Monterrey	Lundell, 1934	Kidney trouble
854. Yerba de la Hueva	unidentified	Durango-Llano Grande near La Ferreria Ferreria	Riley and Trujillo, 1956	Body sores: boil until water turns green; apply liquid to sore areas as needed
855. Yerba del Indio	*Mirabilis froebelii* var. *glabrata* (Behr.) Greene	Baja California-Paipai	Owen, 1963	Bruises and wounds: make tea from root and drink for internal bruises

856. Yerba Jonequil	_Heimia salicifolia_ (H.B.K.) Link	Valley of Mexico-Tepotzlan	Redfield, 1928	Rheumatism: grind up in alcohol and apply very hot
857. Yerba del Lobo (also called Raiz del Lobo)	_Helenium Hoopesii_ Gray	New Mexico-Spanish	Van Der Eerden, 1948	Parturition (to hasten delivery): take powdered root. Laxative: mix powdered root with brandy or whiskey.
	H. Hoopesii Gray	New Mexico-Spanish	Ford, 1966	Internal bruises: grind and drink with water (3)
	H. Hoopesii Gray	New Mexico-Spanish	Curtin, 1947	Rheumatism: rub dry, ground roots on afflicted parts. Pains in ribs and shoulders (from colds or pneumonia): rub dry root or apply mixture of pulverized root and whiskey or water. Stomach trouble: chew root or boil in water and drink. Fever: make tea from root and drink. Colic (infants): use to make poultice with colláile, oshá, altamisa de la sierra, cinnamon, cloves, nutmeg, and ginger; boil in water, strain, and

Spanish Name	Botanical Name	Location	Reference	Use
				use liquid with cornmeal to make paste; spread on patient and cover with cloth.
	Helenium sp.	New Mexico-Spanish	Shulman and Smith, 1962	Toothache: squeeze gummy excrescence of blossom and put on cotton; apply to tooth.
	H. Hoopesii Gray		Kearney and Peebles, 1951	This plant contains dugaldim, a toxic glucoside which causes spewing sickness in sheep
	unidentified	Chihuahua-Juarez	Ford and Ford, 1965	Cough (8)
858. Yerba Mála	Cuscuta curta Engelm.	New Mexico-Spanish	Curtin, 1947	See Cuscuta
859. Yerba de la Mala Mujer	Brickellia reniformis A. Gray	New Mexico-Spanish	Curtin, 1947	Toothache: boil plant and place in mouth
860. Yerba de Mal del Ojo	unidentified	Durango-Rio Grande near La Ferreria	Riley and Trujillo, 1956	Conjunctivitis: boil leaves and use solution for eyedrops

861. Yerba Mansa (also called Yerba del Manso)	<u>Anemopsis</u> <u>californica</u> (Nutt.) Hook. and Arn.	New Mexico-Tewa	Robbins, et al, 1916	Stomachache: drink hot decoction
	<u>Anemopsis</u> <u>californica</u> Hook. and Arn.	New Mexico-Spanish	Curtin, 1947	Abrasions, burns, sores (men or animals): apply root as powder, in a tea, or as a poultice. Sore throat: add ground to water and gargle. Ulcerated gums: apply crushed root. Piles: make ointment with Punche. Stomach trouble and colic (in children): boil roots and give red liquid to drink. Blood purification: take decoction. Digestive upsets, treatment of mucus membrane: take decoction. Dysentery: take powdered root in water. Dysentery (bleeding): combine ground root with raw egg and drink.
	<u>Anemopsis</u> <u>californica</u> (Nutt.) Hook. and Arn.	New Mexico-Spanish	Shulman and Smith, 1962	"Ills resulting from war wounds": boil root with sugar, take before breakfast for a month. Toothache: grind, mix

Spanish Name	Botanical Name	Location	Reference	Use
				with cow fat. *Pujos* (tenesmus): grind, eat in an egg passed through water without salt.
	Anemopsis californica (Nutt.) Hook. and Arn.	New Mexico-Spanish	Ford, 1966	Diarrhea: take as tea. (1) Stomachache: same as above. (5)
(also called Bavisa)	*Anemopsis californica* (Nutt.) Hook. and Arn.	Chihuahua-Juarez	Jones, 1932	Boils: use infusion as wash
	Anemopsis californica (Nutt.) Hook. and Arn.	Chihuahua-Juarez	Ford and Ford, 1965	Sores: use to wash
	Anemopsis californica (Nutt.) Hook. and Arn.	North Mexico	Lumholtz, 1912	Colds, coughs, indigestion: use roots. Wounds, swellings: use roots. Chewing: as tobacco.
	Anemopsis californica (Nutt.) Hook. and Arn.	North Mexico-Yaqui	Holden, et al, 1936	Cuts and bruises: beat to a pulp, mix with rosemary, Yerba Colorado, and Alucema seeds to form a paste to apply
	Anemopsis californica (Nutt.) Hook. and Arn.	Arizona, Sonora, Southern California	Palmer, 1878	Venereal sores: apply powdered root. Cuts: apply powdered root. Swellings: apply wilted leaves.

	Anemopsis californica (Nutt.) Hook. and Arn.	California-Spanish	Curtin, 1947	Swellings: use wilted leaves as poultice. Rheumatism: use as wash or poultice.
	Anemopsis californica (Nutt.) Hook. and Arn.	California-Spanish	Carter, 1947	Sores: use for wash or as poultice
	Anemopsis californica (Nutt.) Hook. and Arn.	California-Spanish	Fearn, 1909	Rheumatism: use as wash or poultice. Blood purifier: take tea made from root. Cuts and sores: take as tea. Swellings: use wilted leaves.
	Anemopsis californica (Nutt.) Hook. and Arn.	California-Spanish	Lloyd, 1914	Malaria: use juice from root. Diarrhea and dysentery.
	Anemopsis californica (Nutt.) Hook. and Arn.	Baja California-Kiliwa	Meigs, 1939	Cough or catarrh: take decoction of root. Headache: put fresh leaves on temple.
	Anemopsis californica (Nutt.) Hook. and Arn.	Baja California-Paipai	Owen, 1963	Colds: take tea of powdered root. Frío: drink tea; use in massage; or inhale fumes.
862. Yerba Mate	*Ilex* sp.	New Mexico-Spanish	Ford, 1966	Beverage: tea

Spanish Name	Botanical Name	Location	Reference	Use
863. Yerba Mora	Solanum pterocaulon Dun. (S. nigrum)	San Luís Potosí-Charcas	Whiting, 1934	Espanto (fright): grind leaf and take juice of unripe fruit (?). Skin inflammations: use ripe (black) fruit.
	Solanum pterocaulon	Nueva Leon-Monterrey	Lundell, 1934	Medicinal herb
	S. nigrum	Valley of Mexico-Tepepan	Madsen, 1965	Chincula (hot illness of a baby): for recipe, see Pata de Leon
	unidentified	Durango-La Ferreria	Riley and Trujillo, 1956	Mashed finger: apply fresh plant or dry powdered plant moistened with water.
	unidentified	Durango-El Torreón near La Ferreria	Riley and Trujillo, 1956	Tranquilizer (for depression?): add water to leaves, beat with a beater, strain; drink before meals for 8 days
864. Yerba de la Muela	unidentified	Chihuahua-Tarahumar	Pennington, 1963b	Toothache: shove stem in caries
865. Yerba de la Mula	Vigueria decurrens	Chihuahua-Tarahumar	Pennington, 1963b	Boils and infections: crush roots and use as poultice

	Eupatorium subintegrum (Greene)	San Luís Potosí-Charcas	Lundell, 1934	Rheumatism
	E. subintegrum (Greene)	Nueva Leon-Monterrey	Lundell, 1934	Medicinal herb
	Lippia sp.	Durango-Llano Grande near La Ferreria	Riley and Trujillo, 1956	Rheumatism and body aches: boil stalks with leaves and use liquid to bathe
	Stevia sp.	Chihuahua-Tarahumar	Bennett and Zingg, 1935	Colic: drink decoction of leaves
866. Yerba de la Negrita	*Sphaeralcea fendleri* A. Gray	New Mexico-Spanish	Curtin, 1947	Tumors (to loosen them): take decoction of fresh leaves. Swelling (to counteract) from insect bites: crush plant, add salt and apply. Headache: use plaster as for bites. Broken bones: make poultice with mashed roots and a little flour. Hair wash (to promote growth): shampoo with mashed leaves and flowers.
	unidentified [mallow]	New Mexico-Spanish	Shulman and Smith, 1962	Massage: use with vaseline for lubricant. Broken bones: use with Punche and Oshá.

Spanish Name	Botanical Name	Location	Reference	Use
				Hair: good to make hair grow.
(Yerba del Negrito)	S. angustifolia (Cav.) G. Don	San Luís Potosí-Charcas	Whiting, 1934	
	S. angustifolia var. cuspidata Gray	San Luís Potosí-Charcas	Whiting, 1934	
	S. hastatula Gray	San Luís Potosí-Charcas	Whiting, 1934	
	unidentified	Chihuahua-Juarez	Ford and Ford, 1965	Sores and cuts (8)
867. Yerba del Negro	Sphaeralcea cuspidata A. Gray	New Mexico-Spanish	Curtin, 1947	Purge: boil piece of root in water and take. Diuretic: drink decoction of plant.
	S. cuspidata Spach	New Mexico-Spanish	Wooton, 1894	
	S. lobata	New Mexico-Spanish	Wooten and Standley, 1915	
	Tournefortia sp.	Durango-San Pedro across river from La Ferreria	Riley and Trujillo, 1956	Corns: grind dry leaves, mix with pork fat; spread on corn and wrap; leave until corn falls off

				(5-6 days)
868. Yerba Nil (?)	*Tagetes lucida* Cav.	West Mexico	Rose, 1899	Scorpion bites. Fever and ague.
869. Yerba Nis (see also Yerba Anis)	*Tagetes florida* Sweet	San Luís Potosí-Charcas	Lundell, 1934	Sweat bath. Food: boil and drink for breakfast tea.
	Tagetes florida Sweet	Nueva Leon-Monterrey	Lundell, 1934	Medicinal herb
870. Yerbanis	*Tagetes* sp.	Durango-Durango	Riley and Trujillo, 1956	Sick headache and stomach-ache: take as tea morning and late at night
	unidentified	Durango-Llano Grande near La Ferreria	Riley and Trujillo, 1956	Headaches: boil upper half of a plant; take hot liquid with aspirin and mescal
871. Yerba Niso	*Artemisia dracunculus*	Baja California-Paipai	Owen, 1963	Stomachache
872. Yerba Nora	*Solanum nigrum* L.	Valley of Mexico-Tepotzlan	Redfield, 1928	Purge: boil with Tet-zotzo (*Bonplandia*); Yerba de San José (*Verbena*) may be added. Inflammations and swellings: boil, mix with alcohol and apply. Fevers: use the above as a wash.

Spanish Name	Botanical Name	Location	Reference	Use
873. Yerba del Oso (also called Raiz del Oso)	*Heracleum lanatum* Michx.	New Mexico-Spanish	Curtin, 1947	Rheumatic pains and tremors in the heart: grind roots and apply powder or mix with lard and rub on; or boil roots and bathe afflicted parts. Diphtheric throat: grind roots, place in paper tube and blow into throat; place root powder in water and use as gargle. Teeth (to tighten): rub powder on gums. Fever: apply root powder to entire body. Paralysis: bathe in solution of the entire plant.
874. Yerba de Pajaro	unidentified	Durango-La Ferreria	Riley and Trujillo, 1956	Dysentery: boil in water until tinted; take as needed each day for 9 days. (Can mix with Lengua de Vaca and Marsaquite.)
875. Yerba Parda	*Helianthus ciliaris* DC.	New Mexico-Spanish	Wooton, 1894	
876. Yerba del Pasmo	*Baccharis pteronioides*	Arizona	Kearney and Peebles, 1964	

	B. glutinosa	Chihuahua-Tarahumar	Pennington, 1963b	See Jarilla del Río
	Aster intricatus	Chihuahua-Tepehuán	Pennington, 1963a	Bruises and wounds: use plant to prepare poultice
	(H) Aplopappus larincofolius A. Gray	Baja California-Paipai	Owen, 1963	Aches, pains, bruises: make tea to use as liniment for massage. Toothache: use tea made from green leaves as mouthwash. Wounds: boil leaves and use to bathe. Frío: with Gobernadora and Yerba Santa make tea to use for massage. Menstrual difficulties: take tea made from leaves when stoppage is due to Frío. Colds. Swollen members. Abortion (to induce).
	Waltheria americana	Chihuahua-Tepehuán	Pennington, 1963a	Wounds and inflammations: boil plant and use liquid as a lotion
877. Yerba del Pasmo de la Sierra	Brickellia laciniata	Chihuahua-Tepehuán	Pennington, 1963a	Swelling and inflammation: crush whole plant and apply as poultice

Spanish Name	Botanical Name	Location	Reference	Use
878. Yerba del Peco	Actaea arguta Nutt.	New Mexico-Spanish	Curtin, 1947	Rheumatic limbs: for recipe see Punche. Neuralgia: for recipe see Trementina de Piñon. Diarrhea and vomiting: roast seeds, pulverize and put a pinch on a soft boiled egg and eat.
879. Yerba de la Peña (also called Yerba de la Piedra)	[Gray Lichen or moss]	New Mexico-Spanish	Curtin, 1947	Pyorrhea: rub on gums. Sores or injuries: grind and apply.
880. Yerba del Pescado	Polygonum pensylvanicum	Chihuahua-Tarahumar	Pennington, 1963b	Fish poison
	unidentified	Valley of Mexico-Tepotzlan	Field, 1953	Scratches, pimples, spots: apply paste of pulverized herb and lemon juice.
	unidentified	New México-Spanish	Curtin, 1947	Stomachache: eat leaves
881. Yerba de la Piedra	[Grey Lichen or moss]	New Mexico-Spanish	Curtin, 1947	See Yerba de la Peña
882. Yerba del Pinacate	Cassia Wislizeni Gray	San Luís Potosí-Charcas	Whiting, 1934	

883. Yerba del Pino	Pinus sp. [yellow pine]	New Mexico-Spanish	Shulman and Smith, 1962	Beverage: boil needles and drink with lemon juice
884. Yerba del Piojo	Tephrosia nicaraguenis	Chihuahua-Tepehuán	Pennington, 1963a	Fleas (on humans and animals): prepare lotion by soaking entire plant for a few minutes
885. Yerba del Piojo de los Puercos	unidentified	Chihuahua-Tepehuán	Pennington, 1963a	Fleas (on humans and animals): crush and apply as poultice
886. Yerba de la Pulga	Dalea sp.	Chihuahua-Tepehuán	Pennington, 1963a	Fleas (on humans): crush leaves for poultice
887. Yerba de la Quintana	Aplopappus spinulosus	New Mexico-Spanish	Curtin, 1947	Abcesses or swelling of face and neck: mash plant with a little salt and place in mouth where pain exists
888. Yerba sin Raiz	Cuscuta curta Engelm.	New Mexico-Spanish	Curtin, 1947	See Cuscuta
889. Yerba Rasposa	Tournefortia densiflora Mart. and Gal.	Valley of Mexico-Tepotzlan	Redfield, 1928	Blisters: rub on leaves
	unidentified	Valley of Mexico-Tepotzlan	Field, 1953	Kidney troubles: take decoction. To increase milk in nursing mothers: take decoction. Blisters: rub on.

Spanish Name	Botanical Name	Location	Reference	Use
890. Yerba de la Sangre (also called Sangre de Cristo)	*Berberis repens* Lindl.	New Mexico-Spanish	Curtin, 1947	Anemia: boil leaves and drink tea twice daily. Menstruation (to stimulate): boil leaves, drink early in morning before eating. Blood purification: boil leaves or roots and drink tepid tea. Anti-syphilitic, diuretic, laxative: take tea from roots.
891. Yerba de San Ignacio	unidentified	Zacatecas-Zacatecas	Riley and Trujillo, 1956	Purgative: pulverize interior of seed, add to water and take
892. Yerba de San José	*Verbena polystachya* H.B.K.	Valley of Mexico-Tepotzlan	Redfield, 1928	Fever: for recipe see Alta Reina. Purge: for recipe see Yerba Nora.
893. Yerba de San Pedro	unidentified	Chihuahua-Tarahumar	Pennington, 1963b	See Vara Blanca
894. Yerba Santa	*Eriodictyon agustifolium* Nutt.	Baja California-Paipai	Owen, 1963	Skin eruptions: boil leaves with Chamiso Blanco and wash irritations; or grind dry leaves and apply. Frío: for recipe see Yerba del Pasmo.

				Stiff neck: tie leaves around neck. Sore throat: make leaves into tea. Aches, bruises, and wounds: heat leaves and apply to affected areas. Coughs and colds: boil leaves and drink.
895. Yerba de Santa Getrudes	unidentified	Durango-Rio Grande near La Ferreria	Riley and Trujillo, 1956	Fever with upset stomach: boil leaves and take in the morning for 5 days
896. Yerba de Santa Maria	<u>Alomia alata</u> Hemsl.	Valley of Mexico-Tepotzlan	Redfield, 1928	Palpitations: grind plant and take in a cup of alcohol with sugar and egg
897. Yerba del Sapo	<u>Franseria tenuifolia</u> Gray	New Mexico-Spanish	Curtin, 1947	This species is considered male. Stomach ulcers in women: mash plant to extract juice, add water and drink. Jumping stomach in women: make a green ball with the plant, wrap in a cloth and place on navel.
	F. confertiflora (DC.) Rydb. and F. acanthicarpa (Hook.) Coville	New Mexico-Spanish	Van Der Eerden, 1948	Parturition (to hasten delivery of baby)

Spanish Name	Botanical Name	Location	Reference	Use
	F. acanthicarpa Hook.	New Mexico-Spanish	Curtin, 1947	This species is considered female. Stomach inflammation in men: grind leaves; mix with salt, asparagus berries; decoct tea, strain and drink. Jumping stomach in men: as for women. To hasten cure of lacerations on backs of burros: sprinkle dry powdered leaves.
(Lleva del Sapo)	Cirsium undulatum (Nutt.) Spreng.	Chihuahua-Juarez	Jones, 1932	Fever: take as tea and use tea to bathe
	Eryngium Carlinae	Chihuahua-Tarahumar	Pennington, 1963b	Styes: bruise flowers and apply as poultice
	E. sp. cf. heterophyllum	Chihuahua-Tarahuan	Pennington, 1963b	Coughs: take tea made from flowers and leaves
	E. Hemsleyanum	Chihuahua-Tepehuán	Pennington, 1963a	Rheumatic pains: take tea made from leaves
	E. wrightii Gray	San Luís Potosí-Charcas	Whiting and Lundell, 1934	Cough: boil in water. Urinary trouble.
	unidentified	New Mexico-Spanish	Ford, 1966	Rheumatism: grind and apply externally

	unidentified	Chihuahua-Juarez	Ford and Ford, 1965	Kidney ailments, venereal disease: boil and take infusion 3 times/day before meals for 5 days. Coughs: take above at night and hot.
(Yerba de Sapo)	Eryngium sp.	Durango-Llano Grande near La Ferreria	Riley and Trujillo, 1956	Coughs: dip leaves into boiling water; take liquid as needed
898. Yerba del Sol	Gaillardia pinnatifida Torr.	New Mexico-Spanish	Curtin, 1947	See Coronilla
899. Yerba del Tomor	Drymaria gracilis C. and S.	San Luís Potosí-Charcas	Whiting, 1934	"Tomor" or swelling on hand or foot: boil in water and use to treat
900. Yerba del Torro	Zinnia linearis Benth.	Western Mexico-Jalisco	Rose, 1899	Stomach pains: make tea from stems
901. Yerba del Transito	unidentified	Durango-Llano Grande near La Ferreria	Riley and Trujillo, 1956	(Rheumatic ?) pains around waist: grind and mix with cooking oil and rub on affected part of body
902. Yerba de la Tusa	Lepachys tagetes A. Gray	New Mexico-Spanish	Curtin, 1947	Red pustules (all over body): boil plant and use liquid to bathe; wrap in sheet and go to bed. Rheumatism: boil plant and use to bathe. Toothache: place powdered

Spanish Name	Botanical Name	Location	Reference	Use
				dry root on tooth to reduce throbbing.
903. Yerba de la Vaca	*Brickellia californica* A. Gray	Baja California-Paipai	Owen, 1963	Coughs and colds: boil leaves or piece of bark in water. Influenza: make tea of leaves. Fever.
904. Yerba del Vaso	*Encelia farinosa* Gray	Southwestern United States	Beal, 1943	See Incienso
905. Yerba del Venado	*Porphyllum gracile* Benth.	Arizona	Kearney and Peebles, 1964	Deer and cattle relish it
	P. gracile Benth.	Baja California-Paipai	Owen, 1963	Coughs and colds: take tea
	P. filifolium *P. filiforme* Rydb.	San Luís Potosí-Charcas	Lundell, 1934	Constipation
906. Yerba de la Verguenza	*Schrankia potosina* (Britt. and Rose) Standley.	San Luís Potosí-Charcas	Whiting, 1934	"Plant of shame"
907. Yerba de la Víbora	*Gutierrezia tenuis* Greene	New Mexico-	Curtin, 1947	See Collálle

		G. tenuis Greene	New Mexico	Wooton and Standley, 1915	
		G. linoides Greene *G. longifolia* Greene	New Mexico-Tewa	Robbins, et al, 1916	See Collálle
		Zornia diphylla	Chihuahua-Tarahumar	Pennington, 1963b	Fever: take as tea
		Zornia diphylla	Chihuahua-Tepehuán	Pennington, 1963a	Pains from gripe: make tea from entire plant
		Zornia diphylla	Chihuahua-Chihuahua	Zingg, 1932	Colds and fevers: take decoction; adults add to liquor (sotol).
		unidentified	Chihuahua-Juarez	Ford and Ford, 1965	Chills: boil in water and take (8)
		unidentified	Chihuahua-Parral	Riley and Trujillo, 1956	Colds and fevers: boil in water and take
	(Yerba de la Vivora)	*Dyschoriste decumbens* (Gray) Kuntze	San Luís Potosí-Charcas	Lundell, 1934	Constipation: boil and drink
	(Yerba Vivora)	*Dychoriste linearis?* Gray ? *Calophanes linearis?*	Nueva Leon-Monterrey	Lundell, 1934	Snakebite
908.	Yerba de Vibora	*Aplopappus* sp.	Durango-Llano Grande near La Ferreria	Riley and Trujillo, 1956	Snakebite: boil and apply hot, wet plant as poultice; let dry

Spanish Name	Botanical Name	Location	Reference	Use
909. Yerba de la Virgen	*Gaura coccinea* Pursh	New Mexico-Spanish	Curtin, 1947	Rheumatism (muscular): grind or mash (green or dry) plants and rub on limbs
	Stevia stenophylla	Chihuahua-Tepehuán	Pennington, 1963a	Broken bones: use plant to prepare poultice
910. Yerba del Zorillo	*Chenopodium incisium* Poir.	New Mexico-Spanish	Curtin, 1947	Colic in babies: boil fruit in water until wine-colored, strain and give to baby. Menstrual pain: boil plant in water and drink. Rheumatism: soak plants in water and use to bathe.
	Chenopodium sp.	Nueva Leon-Monterrey	Lundell, 1934	Medicinal herb
	? *Croton* sp.	Durango-San Pedro across river from La Ferreria	Riley and Trujillo, 1956	Whooping cough; boil leaves until water is tinted; take at night for 5 days
911. Yerba de Zorillo Cimarron	*Chenopodium botrys* L.	New Mexico-Spanish	Curtin, 1947	See Yerba del Chivatito
912. Yuca	*Yucca* sp.	New Mexico-Spanish	Curtin, 1947	See Amole

913. Zábila	*Aloe vulgaris*	Valley of Mexico-Tepotzlan	Madsen, 1965	Pain in the lungs (cold illness), backache caused from overwork in fields, from grinding or washing: rub shoulders with piece which has a certain commercial ointment on it
914. Zacate de Burro	unidentified	Chihuahua-Tepehuán	Pennington, 1963a	Stomach upsets: take as tea
915. Zacate Límon (Te; Te Límon)	*Cymbopogon citratus* (DC.) Stapf	Chihuahua-Juarez	Jones, 1932	Food: make tea, use as beverage
916. Zacate Liso	*Muhlenbergia monticola* Buckl.	San Luis Potosi-Charcas	Whiting, 1934	
917. Zanahoria	*Daucus carota* ? [carrots]	New Mexico-Spanish	Shulman and Smith, 1962	Eyes: good for eyes
918. Zapote	*Achras zapota* *Achras* sp.	Chihuahua-Tarahumar	Pennington, 1963b	Food: eat fruit
(Zapote Blanco)	*Casimiroa edulis*	Valley of Mexico-Tepepan	Madsen, 1965	Parturition: new mother whose bones are cold should have bath in Agua de Romero, for recipe see Tepozan

Spanish Name	Botanical Name	Location	Reference	Use
919. Zarza (also called Sarsa del Campo)	Humulus lupulus neomexicanus Nels. and Ckll.	New Mexico-Spanish	Curtin, 1947	Swollen limbs from dropsy: boil flowers in water and use solution to bathe; then go to bed to induce sweating. Paralysis: as above. Rheumatism: for recipe see Coronilla. Blood: take tea. Food: use to make bread rise.
	Humulus sp. [wild hops hemp family]	New Mexico-Spanish	Shulman and Smith, 1962	Insomnia: use a pillow filled with leaves
920. Zarzagorda	unidentified	Zacatecas-Zacatecas	Riley and Trujillo, 1956	Blood tonic: take decoction of boiled root, 3 times/day for 9 days. Kidney disease: take decoction twice a day for 9 days.
921. Zarza Mora	Rubus idaeus var.	Chihuahua-Tarahumar	Pennington, 1963b	Food: eat berries
922. Zarzaparilla	Humulus lupulus neomexicanus	New Mexico-Spanish	Curtin, 1947	See Zarza
(Sarsaparilla)	Krameria pauciflora DC.	Nueva Leon-Monterrey	Lundell, 1934	Blood tonic. Infected gums (to clean) and for bad teeth.

923. Zarzilla	*Erigeron flagellaris*	New Mexico-Spanish	Curtin, 1947	Kidney trouble: use plant to make tea
924. Zorillo	*Choisya* sp. or *Astrophyllum dumosum*	Arizona	Kearney and Peebles. 1964	
		New Mexico	Wooton and Standley, 1915	
925. Zuelda de Zuelda	unidentified	New Mexico-Spanish	Ford, 1966	Broken bones: use to make casts (3)

SUPPLEMENT TO
APPENDIX F

Botanical Name	Location	Reference	Use
<u>Agastache</u> <u>pallida</u>	Chihuahua-Tarahumar	Bennett and Zingg, 1935	Coughs and colds: drink decoction; place pinch of leaves in nostril to clear head
<u>Allium</u> sp.	New Mexico-Spanish	Van der Eerden, 1948	Parturition: to hasten delivery of baby; the mother takes glass of garlic water, eats raw onion, and/or is rubbed all over body with well-cooked (fried) onions mixed with Manzanilla (<u>Matricaria</u> <u>Chamomilla</u>)
<u>Anagallis</u> <u>aryensis</u>	Chihuahua-Tepehuán	Pennington, 1963a	Catarro (influenza): take as tea
<u>Apocynum</u> <u>sibiricum</u> var. <u>salignum</u> Bern. (Greene)	Baja California-Paipai	Owen, 1963	Menstrual difficulties: boil root and drink tea
<u>Arctostaphylos</u> <u>pungens</u> H.B.K.	Chihuahua-Tarahumar	Bennett and Zingg, 1935	Food: eat fruit
<u>Arisolochia</u> <u>brevipes</u>	Chihuahua-Tarahumar	Pennington, 1963b	Intestinal disorders: take decoction of roots and lower stems
<u>Asclepias</u> <u>Linaria</u>	Chihuahua-Tepehuán	Pennington, 1963a	Stomach cramps: use tea of leaves to induce vomiting Purgative: use larger amounts of leaves than above. Headache: apply crushed leaves to temples.
<u>Asclepias</u> sp.	Chihuahua-Tarahumar	Bennett and Zingg, 1935	Purgative: pound and scald roots, cool and strain liquid and drink.

			Venereal disease.
Asclepias sp.	Chihuahua-Tarahumar	Pennington, 1963b	Rheumatism: use crushed, dampened leaves as a poultice
Baccharis sarothroides A. Gray	Arizona-Spanish	Curtin, 1949	Toothache
Bidens bigelovii Gray		Havard, 1885	Soporific, carminative, and tonic: parboil and dry leaves; then make an infusion
Bonplandia geminiflora Cav.	Valley of Mexico-Tepotzlan	Redfield, 1928	Purge: boil with Solanum nigrum L., may also add Verbena polystachya
Borago officinalis	Valley of Mexico-Tepotzlan	Madsen, 1965	Typhus: use leaves and flowers to make tea (with cinnamon)
Bouvardia glaberrima	Chihuahua-Tarahumar	Pennington, 1963b	Heart trouble: decoct stems and leaves
Brickellia sp.	Chihuahua-Chihuahua	Zingg, 1932	Purgative: boil and take decoction
Buddleia cordata	Chihuahua-Tarahumar	Pennington, 1963b	Boils and sores: heat leaves and apply
Buddleia cordata	Chihuahua-Tarahumar	Bennett and Zingg, 1935	Wounds or bruises: warm leaves in ashes and apply hot as a poultice or use plant to prepare an ointment with lard or suet

Botanical Name	Location	Reference	Use
Buddleia sp.	Chihuahua-Tarahumar	Bennett and Zingg, 1935	Fright: magical cure by a shaman; use shavings of stick to make bathing solution and to drink
Caesalpinia mexicana	Chihuahua-Tarahumar	Bennett and Zingg, 1935	Wounds, sores, ulcers: grind dry roots and sprinkle on
Casimiroa edulis Casimiroa sapota	Chihuahua-Tarahumar	Bennett and Zingg, 1935	Fish stupefaction: pound bark and throw into dammed river. Food: eat fruit.
Cheilanthes Kaulfussii	Chihuahua-Tarahumar	Pennington, 1963b	Pulmonary troubles: take tea made from stems and leaves
Cheilanthes tomentosa	Chihuahua-Tarahumar	Pennington, 1963b	Urinary disorders: take tea made from stems and leaves
Chilopsis linearis (Cav.) Sweet		Havard, 1885	Fever: use flowers. Stimulant: for cardiac diseases.
Chromolepsis heterophylla	Chihuahua-Tepehuán	Pennington, 1963a	Navel of infant: use buttons on root to make poultice to apply to infant's navel when umbilical cord is cut
Cirsium mexicanum	Chihuahua-Tepehuán	Pennington, 1963a	Chest pains: take tea of crushed and boiled roots
Cissus sp.	Chihuahua-Tarahumar	Bennett and Zingg, 1935	Fractures: use sticky juice in stems to set broken bones

Crescentia alata	Chihuahua-Tarahumar	Bennett and Zingg, 1935	Food: eat fruit. Colds: mix green fruit with water.
Croton californicus Muell. Arg.	Baja California-Paipai	Owen, 1963	Venereal disease: use root to make tea
Cupressus arizonica	Chihuahua-Tarahumar	Pennington, 1963b	Coughing: use needles to make tea
Dalea polygonoides	Chihuahua-Tarahumar	Pennington, 1963b	Headache: take tea of crushed leaves
Dichondra repens	Chihuahua-Tarahumar	Pennington, 1963b	Swollen legs: use leaves to make hot decoction to bathe legs
Dryopteris normalis	Chihuahua-Tarahumar	Pennington, 1963b	Backache: use washed roots as a poultice. Menstrual pains: make tea of crushed roots.
Dryopteris pilosa	Chihuahua-Tepehuán	Pennington, 1963a	Post-partum hemorrhage: take decoction of crushed roots. Menstrual pains: drink decoction as above.
Ephedra antisyphilitica Meyer	Arizona-Spanish	Russell, 1908	Syphilis remedy
Erigonium fasciculatum ssp. foliolosum (Nutt.) S. Stockes	Baja California-Paipai	Owen, 1963	Dysentery: tea is made with this and a piece of cholla root
Eryngium Rosei	Chihuahua-Tepehuán	Pennington, 1963a	Heart palpitations: take tea

Botanical Name	Location	Reference	Use
Eryngium sp.	Chihuahua-Tarahumar	Bennett and Zingg, 1935	Colds: boil with salt and take. Headache: take decoction and also rub on head.
Erythrina sp.	Chihuahua-Tarahumar	Bennett and Zingg, 1935	Stomachache: grind toasted seeds, mix with warm water and drink
Eupatorium deltoideum	Valley of Mexico-Tepepan	Madsen, 1965	Anger sickness complicated by the eating of mushrooms: use with other "hot" herbs such as Aníse, Cedrón
Eupatorium sp.	Chihuahua-Tarahumar	Bennett and Zingg, 1935	Purgative: use sticky juice of one species. Stomach disorders: grind raw roots and drink with water.
Euphorbia heterophylla L.	Chihuahua-Tarahumar	Bennett and Zingg, 1935	Food: eat bulb on the root. Fever: eat bulb raw or boil for fever.
Eysenhardtia polyatachya	Chihuahua-Tarahumar	Pennington, 1963b	Pain from internal injuries: crush bark and decoct into drink
Fimbristylis sp.	Chihuahua-Tarahumar	Bennett and Zingg, 1935	Colds and pneumonia: use whole plant to make decoction; strain and drink
Garrya veatchii Kell	Baja California-Paipai	Owen, 1963	Wounds and boils
Gnaphalium wrightii	Baja California-Paipai	Owen, 1963	Coughs and colds: make tea

Grindelia squarrosa (Pursh) Dunal	Southern California-Spanish and "Indian"	Palmer, 1878	Colds: drink decoction of plant
Haematoxylum brasiletto	Chihuahua-Tarahumar	Bennett and Zingg, 1935	Jaundice: use wood to made red liquid for bathing
(H)aplopappus venetus var. furfuraceus (Greene) Hall	Baja California-Paipai	Owen, 1963	Wounds
Helianthemum glomeratum	Chihuahua-Tarahumar	Pennington, 1963b	Fever: infuse leaves to make drink. Coughing: same as above.
Hieracium sp.	Chihuahua-Tarahumar	Bennett and Zingg, 1935	Sores, boils, ulcers: powder dried leaves and apply
Hyptis albida	Chihuahua-Tarahumar	Pennington, 1963b	Parturition: to hasten emergence of afterbirth, use leaves to make tea. Earache: make flowers into small wads and place in the ear. Rheumatic pains: crush entire plant and rub on body.
Hyptis emory Torr.	Chihuahua-Tarahumar	Bennett and Zingg, 1935	Parturition: cook flowers, stem, and leaves in water; women in childbirth drink decoction (because it is "very hot")
Iresine interrupta	Valley of Mexico-Tepotzlan	Redfield, 1928	Fever: grind plant and steep with other herbs such as rose leaves,

Botanical Name	Location	Reference	Use
			wine, and coriander and place on the lungs and abdomen.
<u>Jatropha</u> <u>curcas</u>	Chihuahua-Tarahumar	Bennett and Zingg, 1935	Toothache: use milky juice. Bad eyes: use milky juice.
<u>Jatropha</u> <u>macrorhiza</u> Benth.	New Mexico	Havard, 1885	Emetic and purgative: the rhizome available for sale in powdered form in drugstores. Purgative: seeds.
<u>Juniperus</u> <u>pachyphlaea</u>	Chihuahua-Tarahumar	Pennington, 1963b	Coughing: boil needles and take decoction. Sweat baths.
<u>Karwinskia</u> <u>humboldtiana</u>	Chihuahua-Tarahumar	Bennett and Zingg, 1935	Headache: wrap leaves in a cloth and tie around the head
<u>Krameria</u> sp.	Chihuahua-Tarahumar	Pennington, 1963b	Toothache: grind the skin and apply directly or mix with suet
<u>Krameria</u> sp.	Chihuahua-Tarahumar	Bennett and Zingg, 1935	Toothache: grind the skin and apply directly or mix with suet
<u>Krameria</u> <u>grayi</u> Rose and Painter <u>Krameria</u> <u>canescens</u> Gray	New Mexico	Havard, 1885	Dye: use infusion of bark of root to dye leather brownish-red
<u>Larrea</u> <u>tridentata</u> (DC.) Coville	Arizona-Spanish	Riley, 1889	Rheumatic affections: use infusion of leaves for bathing
<u>Larrea</u> <u>tridentata</u> (DC.) Coville	Baja California-Kiliwa	Meigs, 1939	"Slow" blood: drink lukewarm tea made from leaf (and also, give to

			animals)
<u>Larrea tridentata</u> (DC.) Coville	Southwestern United States-Spanish	Havard, 1885	Rheumatic affections: use infusion of branchlets and leaves for bathing
<u>Litsea glaucesens</u>	Chihuahua-Tarahumar	Pennington, 1963b	Stomach disorders: use leaves to make tea
<u>Litsea glaucescens</u>	Chihuahua-Tarahumar and "Mexicans"	Bennett and Zingg, 1935	Colic: take tea (Tarahumar). Beverage: tea ("Mexicans").
<u>Magnolia Schiedeana</u>	Chihuahua-Tepehuán	Pennington, 1963a	Stomach pains: use flowers to prepare tea
<u>Malva parviflora</u>	Chihuahua-Tarahumar	Pennington, 1963b	Sores: mash leaves, mix with ground corn and apply. Purgative: use infusion for enema.
<u>Mascagnia macroptera</u>	Chihuahua-Tarahumar	Pennington, 1963b	Toothache: scrape and bruise bark, mix with animal fat, and apply. Sprains and fractures: use crushed bark as a poultice.
<u>Matelea</u> sp.	Chihuahua-Tarahumar	Pennington, 1963b	Boils: crush roots and use in poultice
<u>Muhlenbergia Porteri</u>	Chihuahua-Tarahumar	Pennington, 1963b	Backache or rheumatic pains: use boiled and mashed roots as a poultice
<u>Nicotiana attenuata</u> Torr.	Baja California-Kiliwa	Meigs, 1939	Cough: smoke in reed tube

Botanical Name	Location	Reference	Use
Nicotiana glauca Graham	Chihuahua-Tarahumar	Bennett and Zingg, 1935	Headache: apply leaves to head
Nicotiana glauca Graham	Chihuahua-Tarahumar	Pennington, 1963b	Headache: heat leaves and apply to head
Papaver rhoeas	Chihuahua-Tepehuán	Pennington, 1963a	Fever (sedative): boil flowers for tea and give to quiet fever-stricken people
Parmelia caperata	Chihuahua-Tarahumar	Pennington, 1963b	Burns: dry, crush, and then dust on burns
Pectis stenophylla	Chihuahua-Tarahumar	Pennington, 1963b	Urinary troubles: make leaves into tea. Colds: inhale vapors from this tea.
Penstemon centranthifolius Benth.	Baja California-Paipai	Owen, 1963	Stomachache and vomiting: drink tea. Diarrhea and dysentery: take tea of whole plant.
Peucephyllum	Baja California-Kiliwa	Meigs, 1939	Swellings and sore feet: use warm brew of leaf for washing body
Pinus arizonica	Chihuahua-Tepehuán	Pennington, 1963a	Fever: crush budding cones on a rock and use to prepare tea. Coughing attacks: tea as above.
Pinus ayacahuite	Chihuahua-Tepehuán	Pennington, 1963a	Wounds (on feet): use gum as a poultice

Pinus ayacahuite	Chihuahua-Tarahumar	Pennington, 1963b	Cough: use needles with Pinus reflexa and Pinus lumholtzii to make tea. Foot infections: heat pitch and use as ointment.
Pinus engelmanni	Chihuahua-Tepehuán	Pennington, 1963a	Influenza (catarro): cook fresh stems and eat. Mash and chew the mature stems.
Pinus leiophylla	Chihuahua-Tepehuán	Pennington, 1963a	Sores: apply gum from the bark
Pinus reflexa	Chihuahua-Tarahumar	Pennington, 1963b	Cough: use needles (with Pinus lumholtzii and Pinus ayacahuite) to make tea. Rheumatism: obtain a crude turpentine by notching trunks; use as rubbing compound. Lung congestion: make a very weak tea from the crude turpentine.
Pisonia capitata	Chihuahua-Tarahumar	Bennett and Zingg, 1935	Fevers: grind leaves with water, put juice obtained in fresh water, and take the decoction warm.
Pithecollobium dulce	Chihuahua-Tarahumar	Bennett and Zingg, 1935	Sore eyes: boil leaves to make a wash
Plumbago scandens	Chihuahua-Tarahumar	Pennington, 1963b	Intestinal disorders: crush roots and branches and use to make tea. Rheumatism: use tea as above.

Botanical Name	Location	Reference	Use
Plumeria acutifolia	Chihuahua-Tarahumar	Bennett and Zingg, 1935	Purgative: pound and grind root (or bark), mix with water, and take
Polypodium aureum?	Valley of Mexico-Tepotzlan	Field, 1953	Liver, gall bladder, and kidney ailments: boil Waltheria americana, add sugar, then add Polypodium
Prunus capuli	Chihuahua-Tarahumar	Pennington, 1963b	Whooping cough and bronchitis: use leaves to make tea
Ptelea trifoliata	Chihuahua-Tarahumar	Bennett and Zingg, 1935	Rheumatism: boil leaves and decoct. Use as a bath or wash for body or face.
Ptelea trifoliata	Chihuahua-Tarahumar	Pennington, 1963b	Rheumatism: make a wash from leaves and roots
Purshia tridentata	Chihuahua-Tarahumer	Pennington, 1963b	Boils: mash leaves and use as a poultice
Quercus arizonica	Chihuahua-Tarahumar	Pennington, 1963b	Sore or inflamed armpits and neck: crush fresh bark and moisten for use as a salve to rub on these areas
Quercus chihuahuensis	Chihuahua-Tarahumar	Pennington, 1963b	Pregnancy: use sap obtained by notching the bark to make tea for use during pregnancy. Heart ailments: take tea as above.
Quercus viminea	Chihuahua-Tarahumar	Pennington, 1963b	Stomach upsets: take decoction made from steeped leaves

Ranunculus sp.	Chihuahua-Tepehuán	Pennington, 1963a	Aching gums: mash roots and apply
Ratibida mexicana	Chihuahua-Tarahumar	Pennington, 1963b	Headaches or colds: pulverize leaves and roots and infuse in hot water; then drink. Sores (festering): pulverize roots and use as a poultice.
Ribes neglectum	Chihuahua-Tarahumar	Pennington, 1963b	Headache: hold leaves upon fore-head or wrap in a rag and tie about head.
Ricinus communis	Chihuahua-Tarahumar	Pennington, 1963b	Inflammations, boils, swollen places, bruises: heat fresh beans and apply, or smear leaves with fat and use as a poultice. Stomach disorders: chew beans.
Salix amygdaloides Anders.?	Mexico?	Havard, 1885	Yellow fever and malaria: crush leaves and use an infusion internally and externally
Salvia mexicana L.	Valley of Mexico-Tepotzlan	Redfield, 1928	Respiratory ailments (e.g. croup in children): make infusion with this, lemon flowers, and Viguiera grammatoglossa DC. and apply to chest
Sambucus mexicana Presl	Arizona (?) "Mexicans"-Pima, Maricopa	Curtin, 1949	Fever: use dried flowers to make tea and drink. Stomachache, colds, sore throat: use flowers to make tea.

Botanical Name	Location	Reference	Use
Sambucus mexicana Presl	Baja California-Kiliwa	Meigs, 1939	Catarrh: drink brew made from white flower
Senecio Hartwegii	Chihuahua-Tarahumar	Pennington, 1963b	Lice or ticks (to kill): crush roots and rub on people or animals
Senecio sp.	Chihuahua-Tarahumar	Bennett and Zingg, 1935	Sores and boils: mix dried plant with water and apply
Solanum diversifolium	Chihuahua-Tarahumar	Pennington, 1935	Rheumatic pains: boil whole plant and rub the liquid on the body. Colds: take above mixture as tea.
Solanum nigrum	Chihuahua-Tarahumar	Bennett and Zingg, 1935	Pneumonia: cook branch and make hot applications to the chest and cold applications to the back
Solanum nigrum	Chihuahua-Tarahumar	Pennington, 1963b	Rheumatic pains: cook leaves, cool, drain, and use as a poultice
Solanum rostratum	Chihuahua-Tarahumar	Pennington, 1963b	Menstruation: use leaves to make tea for women during menstruation
Solanum verbascifolium	Chihuahua-Tarahumar	Pennington, 1963b	Sores: heat leaves and use as a poultice
Solanum verbascifolium	Chihuahua-Tarahumar	Bennett and Zingg, 1935	Wounds or sores: heat leaves in ashes and apply
Solanum sp.	Chihuahua-Tepehuán	Pennington, 1963a	Toothache: crush fresh leaves and place between cheek and gum. Fever: use leaves to prepare tea.

Sphaeralcea ambigua Gray	Baja California-Paipai	Owen, 1963	Skin eruptions: boil leaves and use the tea to wash pimples and blemishes on face and hands of children
Sphaeralcea Fenderli Gray	New Mexico-Spanish	Sergeant, no date	Wave set for hair: use crushed plant
Stemmadenia Palmeri	Chihuahua-Tarahumar	Pennington, 1963b	Styes: use latex as a poultice. Boils and festering sores: pulverize and apply dried latex.
Stevia micrantha Lag.	Valley of Mexico-Tepotzlan	Redfield, 1928	Ailments caused by the evil spirits of the air: boil plant, mix with alcohol and take internally
Stevia salicifolia	Chihuahua-Tarahumar	Pennington, 1963b	Toothache: place stems into caries or chew the root. Sores (caused by worms) on animals: mash leaves and place into sores.
Stevia serrata	Chihuahua-Tarahumar	Pennington, 1963b	Same as above (*Stevia salicifolia*)
Tabebuia Palmeri	Chihuahua-Tarahumar	Pennington, 1963b	Pulmonary disturbances or backaches: take tea of fresh stems and leaves
Tagetes jaliscana	Chihuahua-Tepehuán	Pennington, 1963a	Stomach disorders: use whole plant to make tea
Tagetes lucida	Chihuahua-Tarahumar	Pennington, 1963b	Beverage: use leaves to make weak tea. Internal ailments: use leaves to make strong tea.

Botanical Name	Location	Reference	Use
Tecoma stans (L.) H.B.K.	Valley of Mexico-Tepotzlan	Redfield, 1928	Constipation or indigestion in children: boil with stone of mamey, Senecio sp. (Lechugilla), and saca-sili (unidentified) and drink the resulting infusion
Tephrosia leiocarpa	Chihuahua-Tarahumar	Pennington, 1963b	Fleas, lice, ticks: crush roots and use as a poultice to eliminate these insects from people and animals
Thalictrum Fendleri	Chihuahua-Tarahumar	Pennington, 1963b	Heat prostration or "suffocation": use leaves to make tea or use a decoction of the leaves to rub the patient
Thryallis glauca (Cav.) Kuntze	Valley of Mexico-Tepotzlan	Redfield, 1928	Costumbre Blanca (white menses): boil this plant with Hypericum Pratense Schlecht and two unidentified plants and give to pregnant women suffering from this ailment. "Loosening of the female organs": use with Selaginella cuspidata.
Tillandsia benthamiana	Chihuahua-Tarahumar	Bennett and Zingg, 1935	Purgative: boil plant in water and take the decoction
Tillandsia Karwinskyana	Chihuahua-Tarahumar	Pennington, 1963b	Constipation: use leaves to make tea
Tillandsia sp.	Chihuahua-Tarahumar	Pennington, 1963b	Rheumatic pains: boil leaves to prepare a wash

Tithonia fruticosa	Chihuahua-Tarahumar	Pennington, 1963b	Coughs: crush flower petals and and steep to make drink to take
Tragia ramosa	Chihuahua-Tarahumar	Pennington, 1963b	Heart ailments: use leaves tc make decoction to drink
Trichostemma lanatum Benth.	Southern California-"Mexican" and "Indian"	Palmer, 1878	Hair tonic and dye: use leaves to make strong decoction to apply to hair
Turnera ulmifolia	Chihuahua-Tarahumar	Pennington, 1963b	Diarrhea: drink tea of leaves steeped in very hot water
Verbena sp.	Chihuahua-Tepehuán	Pennington, 1963a	Cuts that will not heal: crush leaves and use to make poultice. Stomach cramps: crush, salt, and eat.
Viguiera grammatoglossa DC.	Valley of Mexico-Tepotzlan	Redfield, 1928	Respiratory disease (e.g. croup): for recipe see Salvia mexicana above
Vitis arizonica	Chihuahua-Tepehuán	Pennington, 1963a	Scratches: use leaves to prepare poultice
Woodsia mexicana	Chihuahua-Tarahumar	Pennington, 1963b	Aches and pains: use leaves to make a decoction

APPENDIX G

BOTANICAL NAME DICTIONARY

This appendix provides an index, arranged by botanical name, to the plants listed elswhere in this volume by Spanish name.

BOTANICAL NAME	PLANT FAMILY	SPANISH NAME
1. *Abronia fragrans* Nutt. ex Hook.	Nyctaginaceae	Lechuguilla
2. *Abutilon trisulcatum* (Jacq.) Urb.	Malvaceae	Malva
3. *Acacia cochliacantha* Humb. & Bonpl. ex Willd.	Leguminosae	Vinola
4. *Acacia constricta* Benth. in A.Gray	Leguminosae	Chaparro Prieto
5. *Acacia cymbispina* Sprague & Riley	Leguminosae	Vinola
6. *Acacia farnesiana* (L.) Willd.	Leguminosae	Binorama; Vinorama; Huisache
7. *Acacia filicioides* (Cav.) Trel.	Leguminosae	Timbre; Timbé
8. *Acacia greggii* A.Gray	Leguminosae	Uña de Gato Patitos
9. *Acacia pennatula* Benth. in Hook.	Leguminosae	Algarroba
10. *Acacia willardiana* Rose	Leguminosae	
11. *Acacia* sp.	Leguminosae	Huisache
12. *Acalypha californica* Benth.	Euphorbiaceae	Yerba Congrena
13. *Acalypha hederacea* Torr.	Euphorbiaceae	Yerba del Cancer
14. *Acalypha lindheimeri* Muell. Arg.	Euphorbiaceae	Yerba del Cancer
15. *Acalypha phleoides* Cav.	Euphorbiaceae	Yerba del Cancer; Yerba de la Hormega
16. *Acer negundo* L.	Aceraceae	Nogal
17. *Achillea lanulosa* Nutt.	Compositae	Plumajillo
18. *Achras zapota* L.	Sapotaceae	Zapote

BOTANICAL NAME	PLANT FAMILY	SPANISH NAME
19. Actaea arguta Nutt.	Ranunculaceae	Yerba del Peco
20. Acthaetogeron sp.	Compositae	Mal de Ojase
21. Adenostoma sparsifolium Torr. in Emory	Rosaceae	Chamiso Colorado
22. Adiantum capillus-veneris L.	Polypodiaceae	Celantillo de Ojo de Agua; Culantrillo; Silantriyo
23. Agastache pallida (Lindl.) Cory.	Labiatae	
24. Agave americana L.	Amaryllidaceae	
25. Agave bovicornuta Gentry	Amaryllidaceae	Sabila
26. Agave lecheguilla Torr.	Amaryllidaceae	Lechuguilla; Amole
27. Agave palmeri Engelm. A. parryi Engelm.	Amaryllidaceae	Amole
28. Agave perplexans Trel.	Amaryllidaceae	Lechuguilla Mansa
29. Agave sp.	Amaryllidaceae	Pita; Mescal; Amole Pulque
30. Ageratum sp.	Compositae	Amula
31. Allium cepa L.	Liliaceae	Cebolla
32. Allium cernuum Roth A. recurvatum Rydb.	Liliaceae	Cebollita del Campo
33. Allium sativum L.	Liliaceae	Ajo
34. Allium scaposum Benth. A. kunthii G. Don	Liliaceae	Sevollita del Campo
35. Algae		Lama del Agua
36. Alnus incana (L.) Moench	Betulaceae	
37. Aloe vulgaris Lam.	Liliaceae	Zabila

BOTANICAL NAME	FAMILY	SPANISH NAME
38. Aloe sp.	Liliaceae	Savila
39. Alomia alata Hemsl.	Compositae	Yerba de Santa Maria
40. Aloysia triphylla (L'Hér.) Britton	Verbenaceae	Cedrón
41. Alternanthera repens (L.) Ktze.	Amaranthaceae	Tianguis; Tianguis-pepetla
42. Amaranthus blitoides S.Wats. A. graecizans L.	Amaranthaceae	Chile Puerco; Quelite
43. Amaranthus cruentus L. A. paniculatus L.	Amaranthaceae	Alegría; Bledo; Quelite Morado
44. Amaranthus hybridus L.	Amaranthaceae	Quelite Morado
45. Amaranthus leucocarpus S. Wats.	Amaranthaceae	Cinco de Manyo
46. Amaranthus powellii S. Wats	Amaranthaceae	Quelites Yus; Quelites Colorado Yus
47. Amaranthus retroflexus L. A. chlorostachys Willd. A. blitoides S. Wats.	Amaranthaceae	Calite de Agua; Quelite
48. Amoreuxia palmatifida Moc. & Sessé ex DC.	Cochlospermaceae	Sayas
49. Anagallis arvensis L.	Primulaceae	Coralillo
50. Anemopsis californica (Nutt.) Hook. & Arn.	Saururaceae	Yerba Mansa; Yerba del Manso (Manzo); Yerba del Manzo; Hoja de Babisa; Bavisa
51. Anethum graveolens L.	Umbelliferae	Neldo
52. Angelica sp.	Umbelliferae	Angélica

BOTANICAL NAME	FAMILY	SPANISH NAME
53. *Anoda acerifolia* (Zucc.) DC. *A. hastata* Cav.	Malvaceae	Altea
54. *Anogra* see *Oenothera*		
55. *Anthemis* sp.	Compositae	Manzanilla
56. *Aplopappus* see *Haplopappus*		
57. *Apocynum lividum* Greene in Tidest. & Kittell	Apocynaceae	Lechuguilla
58. *Apocynum sibiricum* Jacq., var. *salignum* (Greene) Fernald	Apocynaceae	
59. *Apocynum* sp.	Apocynaceae	
60. *Arbutus arizonica* (A. Gray) Sarg. *A. glandulosa* Mart. & Gal.	Ericaceae	Madroño
61. *Arctostaphylos pungens* H.B.K.	Ericaceae	Manzanita; Manzanilla
62. *Arctostaphylos uva-ursi* (L.) Spreng.	Ericaceae	Coralillo; Manzanita
63. *Argemone ochroleuca* Sweet	Papaveraceae	Cardo
64. *Argemone platyceras* Link & Otto, var. *hispida* (Gray) Prain *A. hispida* Gray	Papaveraceae	Cardo Santo
65. *Argemone* sp.	Papaveraceae	Chicalote
66. *Ariocarpus fissuratus* (Engelm.) Schum. in Engl. & Prantl.	Cactaceae	Peyote Cimarrón
67. *Aristolochia anguicida* Jacq. *A. foetida* H.B.K.	Aristolochiaceae	Indio
68. *Aristolochia brevipes* Benth.	Aristolochiaceae	Santa María
69. *Aristolochia* sp.	Aristolochiaceae	Artistolochia; Huaco
70. *Artemisia dracunculus* L.	Compositae	Yerba Niso
71. *Artemisia filifolia* Torr.	Compositae	Romerillo

BOTANICAL NAME	FAMILY	SPANISH NAME
72. Artemisia franserioides Greene	Compositae	Altamisa de la Sierra
73. Artemisia frigida Willd.	Compositae	Estafiate
74. Artemisia gnaphalodes Nutt. A. rhizomata A. Nels.	Compositae	Mariola
75. Artemisia ludoviciana Nutt.	Compositae	Rosabari
76. Artemis ludoviciana Nutt. A. mexicana Willd. ex Spreng.	Compositae	Estafiate; Istafiate; Agenjo
77. Artemisia mexicana Willd. ex Spreng. ? or A. ludoviciana Nutt., ssp. mexicana (Willd. ex Spreng.) Keck	Compositae	Alcanfor
78. Artemisia redolens A. Gray	Compositae	Anisote
79. Artemisia tridentata Nutt. A. bigelovii A. Gray	Compositae	Chamiso Hediondo; Estafiate
80. Artemisia vulgaris L.	Compositae	Ajenjo
81. Artemisia sp.	Compositae	Altamisa
82. Arundo donax L.	Gramineae	Caña de Castilla; Carrizo
83. Asclepias capricornu Woodson Asclepiodora decumbens (Nutt.) Gray	Asclepiadaceae	Inmortal
84. Asclepias galioides H.B.K.	Asclepiadaceae	Lechones
85. Asclepias hypoleuca (A. Gray) Woodson	Asclepiadaceae	Venado Oreja
86. Asclepias latifolia (Torr.) Raf.	Asclepiadaceae	Lechones
87. Asclepias linaria Cav.	Asclepiadaceae	
88. Asclepias mexicana Cav.	Asclepiadaceae	Lechona

BOTANICAL NAME	FAMILY	SPANISH NAME
89. *Asclepias quinquedentata* A. Gray	Asclepiadaceae	Contrayerba de la Sierra
90. *Asclepias setosa* Benth.	Asclepiadaceae	Tarumarra
91. *Asclepias speciosa* Torr.	Asclepiadaceae	Lecheros
92. *Asclepias tuberosa* L.	Asclepiadaceae	Inmortal
93. *Asphodelus fistulosus* L.	Liliaceae	Estrella del Norte
94. *Asplenium monanthes* L.	Polypodiaceae	Calaguala
95. *Aster intricatus* (A. Gray) Blake	Compositae	Yerba del Pasmo
96. *Aster spinosus* Benth.	Compositae	Scoba
97. *Astrophyllum dumosum* (Torr.) A. Gray see *Choisya* sp.	Rutaceae	Zorilla
98. *Atriplex canescens* (Pursh) Nutt.	Chenopodiaceae	Chamiso; Chamiza; Cenizo; Chamiso Blanco
99. *Aulosperum* see *Cymopterus*		
100. *Avena fatua* L.	Granineae	Trigillo Loco
101. *Baccharis glutinosa* Pers.	Compositae	Yerba del Pasmo; Vara Dulce; Jar-illa; Juatamote; Batamote
102. *Baccharis pteronioides* DC.	Compositae	Yerba de Pasmo
103. *Baccharis sarothroides* A. Gray	Compositae	
104. *Baccharis viminea* DC.	Compositae	Yerba de Flecha; Jarilla
105. *Baccharis* sp.	Compositae	Pasmo;Popote

BOTANICAL NAME	FAMILY	SPANISH NAME
106. *Berberis fremontii* Torr.	Berberidaceae	Palo Amarillo
107. *Berberis repens* Lindl.	Berberidaceae	Yerba de la Sangre; Sangre de Cristo
108. *Berlandiera lyrata* Benth., var. *macrophylla* A. Gray	Compositae	Coronilla
109. *Berlandiera* sp.	Compositae	Coronilla
110. *Bidens aurea* (Ait.) Sherff	Compositae	Te de Coral
111. *Bidens bigelovii* A. Gray	Compositae	Acetilla
112. *Bidens ferulaefolia* DC.	Compositae	Te
113. *Bidens leucantha* (L.) Willd.	Compositae	Laceta; Aceitilla
114. *Bidens* sp.	Compositae	Picaro
115. *Bocconia arborea* S. Wats.	Papaveraceae	Gediondillo; Palo del Diablo
116. *Boerhaavia mutabilis* R. Br. *B. repens* L.	Nyctaginaceae	Saranda
117. *Bonplandia geminiflora* Cav.	Polemoniaceae	
118. *Borago officinalis* L.	Boraginaceae	Boraja; Borraja
119. *Bougainvillea spectabilis* Willd.	Nyctaginaceae	Bogambilia
120. *Bouteloua gracilis* (H.B.K.) Griffiths	Gramineae	Artizuilla or Artiguilla
121. *Bouvardia glaberrima* Engelm. in Wisliz.	Rubiaceae	
122. *Bouvardia* sp.	Rubiaceae	Trompetilla
123. *Brassica campestris* L.	Cruciferae	Mostaza
124. *Brassica eruca* L. *Eruca sativa* Mill.	Cruciferae	Saramago

BOTANICAL NAME	FAMILY	SPANISH NAME
125. *Brickellia californica* (Torr. & Gray) A. Gray	Compositae	Yerba de la Vaca
126. *Brickellia laciniata* A. Gray	Compositae	Yerba del Pasmo de la Sierra
127. *Brickellia reniformis* A. Gray	Compositae	Yerba de la Mala Mujer
128. *Brickellia* sp. *Coleosanthus* sp.	Compositae	Peston; Prodigiosa
129. *Buddleia americana* L.	Loganiaceae	Tepozan
130. *Buddleia cordata* H.B.K.	Loganiaceae	
131. *Buddleia scordioides* H.B.K.	Loganiaceae	Salvía; Escobilla; Escobillo; Salvilla; Suelda
132. *Buddleia sessiliflora* H.B.K.	Loganiaceae	Teposán; Lengua de Vaca
133. *Buddleia tomentella* Standl.	Loganiaceae	Palo Cenizo
134. *Buddleia* sp.	Loganiaceae	
135. *Bursera grandifolia* (Schlecht.) Engl.	Burseraceae	Palo Mulato
136. *Bursera pubescens* Standl. *Elaphrim pubescens* Schlecht.	Burseraceae	Zarzafras
137. *Cacalia decomposita* A. Gray	Compositae	Matariqui; Matarique
138. *Caesalpinia platyloba* S. Wats.	Leguminosae	Palo Colorado
139. *Caesalpinia pulcherrima* (L.) Swartz	Leguminosae	Flor de Camaron; Tavachin
140. *Calamus draco* Willd.	Palmaceae	Sangre de Venado
141. *Calea zacatechichi* Schlecht.	Compositae	Prodigiosa

BOTANICAL NAME	FAMILY	SPANISH NAME
142. Calliandra californica Benth.	Leguminosae	Tabardillo
143. Calliandra eriophylla Benth.	Leguminosae	Brasilillo
144. Calliandra humilis Benth., var. reticulata (A. Gray) Benson	Leguminosae	Sensitiva
145. Calocarpum mammosum L. Pierre in Urban	Sapotaceae	Hueso de Mamey
146. Cannabis sativa L.	Moraceae	Marijuana
147. Capriola dactylon Ktze.	Gramineae	Pata de Gallo
148. Capsicum annuum L., var. baccatum (L.) Ktze. C. baccatum L.	Solanaceae	Chillipiquin
149. Capsicum annuum L.	Solanaceae	Chile; Chili
150. Capsicum annuum L. C. frutescens	Solanaceae	Chiltipiquin
151. Cardiospermum halicacabum L.	Sapindaceae	Rayo
152. Carthamus tinctorius L.	Compositae	Azafrán
153. Carum petroselinum L. Petroselinum crispum Nym.	Umbelliferae	Perejil
154. Casimiroa edulis Llave & Lex.	Rutaceae	Zapote Blanco
155. Casimiroa sapota Oerst.	Rutaceae	
156. Cassia bauhinioides A. Gray	Leguminosae	Pata de Ves; Pata de Res
157. Cassia fistula L.	Leguminosae	Cañafistola
158. Cassia laevigata Willd.	Leguminosae	Guajillo
159. Cassia skinneri Benth.	Leguminosae	Paraca
160. Cassia wislizenii A. Gray	Leguminosae	Yerba de Pinacate

BOTANICAL NAME	FAMILY	SPANISH NAME
161. *Cassia* sp.	Leguminosae	Hoja de Sen
162. *Castela texana* (Torr. & Gray) Rose	Simarubaceae	Visvirinda
163. *Castilleja arvensis* Cham. & Schlecht.	Scrophulariaceae	Saumyate
164. *Castilleja integra* A. Gray *C. linariaefolia* Benth.	Scrophulariaceae	Flor de Santa Rita
165. *Castilleja* sp.	Scrophulariaceae	Chupon; Varas de San José; Yerba de Apache
166. *Ceiba acuminata* (S. Wats.) Rose	Bombacaceae	Pochote
167. *Ceiba pentandra* (L.) Gaertn.	Bombacaceae	Cabellito de Angel
168. *Celtis pallida* Torr.	Ulmaceae	Capulin; Granjén
169. *Celtis reticulata* Torr.	Ulmaceae	Palo Duro
170. *Celtis* sp.	Ulmaceae	Palo Blanco
171. *Cenchrus incertus* M. A. Curtis *C. pauciflorus* Benth.	Gramineae	Roseta; Sacate Cochinillo
172. *Cenchrus tribuloides* L.	Gramineae	Roseta
173. *Centaurea americana* Nutt.	Compositae	Flor de Cardo Santo
174. *Centaurea rothrockii* Greenman	Compositae	Cardo Santo
175. *Cercocarpus montanus* Raf.	Rosaceae	Palo Duro
176. *Chaptalia seemannii* Hemsl.	Compositae	Telempalcate
177. *Cheilanthes kaulfussii* Kunze	Polypodiaceae	
178. *Cheilanthes tomentosa* Link	Polypodiaceae	

BOTANICAL NAME	FAMILY	SPANISH NAME
179. Chenopodium album L.	Chenopodiaceae	Quelite Salado; Quelites Salados; Calite
180. Chenopodium ambrosioides L.	Chenopodiaceae	Pazote; Hipazote; Epazote Ipazote; Epazote de Comer; Pasote de Comer; Quelite
181. Chenopodium ambrosioides L., var. anthelminticum (L.) A. Gray	Chenopodiaceae	Pazote
182. Chenopodium botrys L.	Chenopodiaceae	Yerba del Chivatito; Yerba de Zorrillo Cimarrón
183. Chenopodium incisum Poir.	Chenopodiaceae	Ipazote del Zorrillo; Yerba del Zorrillo
184. Chenopodium sp.	Chenopodiaceae	Quelite; Ipasote Sarrillo; Yerba Zorrillo; Chichiquelite
185. Chilopsis linearis (Cav.) Sw. var.	Bignoniaceae	Sauce
186. Chilopsis linearis (Cav.) Sw. C. saligna D. Don.	Bignoniaceae	
187. Chimaphila maculata (L.) Pursh	Ericaceae	
188. Chlorophora sp.	Urticaceae	Mora
189. Choisya sp.	Rutaceae	Sorilla or Zorrillo

BOTANICAL NAME	FAMILY	SPANISH NAME
190. Chorizanthe fimbriata Nutt.	Polygonaceae	Bachata; Yerba del Empacho
191. Chromolepis heterophylla Benth.	Compositae	
192. Chrysactinia mexicana A. Gray	Compositae	Damiana; Yerba de San Nicolas; San Nicholas
193. Chrysanthemum balsamita L.	Compositae	Romero de Castilla
194. Chrysanthemum indicum L.	Compositae	Crisanta; Crisantemo
195. Chrysanthemum parthenium (L.) Bernh.	Compositae	Alta Mesa
196. Chrysanthemum parthenium Pers.	Compositae	Altamisa Mexicana
197. Chrysothamnus graveolens (Nutt.) Greene	Compositae	Chamiso Cimarrón; Chamiso Blanco; Mariquilla
198. Cinchona sp.	Rubiaceae	Copalquîn
199. Cinnamomum sp.	Lauraceae	Canela en Raja; Alcan-for
200. Cirsium mexicanum DC.	Compositae	
201. Cirsium undulatum (Nutt.) Spreng.	Compositae	Cardo Santo; Yerba del Sapo
202. Cirsium undulatum "Gray"	Compositae	Flor de Cardo Santo
203. Cirsium sp.	Compositae	Cardo Santo
204. Cissus sp.	Vitaceae	
205. Citrus aurantifolia (Christm.) Swing.	Rutaceae	Flor de Limon

BOTANICAL NAME		FAMILY	SPANISH NAME
206.	Citrus limonia Osbeck	Rutaceae	Limon
207.	Citrus medica	Rutaceae	Cidra
208.	Citrus sp.	Rutaceae	Azar de Naranjo
209.	Clematis drummondii Torr. & Gray	Ranunculaceae	Barba de Chivo
210.	Cleome serrulata Pursh	Capparidaceae	Guaco
211.	Cleome sp.	Capparidaceae	Alcachopa
212.	Clethra (mexicana DC. ?)	Clethraceae	Flor de Tilia (de Bola)
213.	Cnidoscolus angustidens Torr.	Euphorbiaceae	Mala Mujer
214.	Cocos nucifera L.	Palmaceae	Barba de Coco
215.	Coldenia greggii (Torr.) Gray	Boraginaceae	Yerba de la Cachucha
216.	Coleosanthus see Brickellia		
217.	Condalia spathulata A. Gray	Rhamnaceae	Teconblate
218.	Cordia boissieri DC.	Boraginaceae	Flor de Nacahuila
219.	Cordia sp.	Boraginaceae	Pala Anaca-huite; Trompillo
220.	Coreopsis tinctoria Nutt.	Compositae	Berros
221.	Coriandrum sativum L.	Umbelliferae	Culantro; Cilantro
222.	Cosmos parviflorus (Jacq.) Pers.	Compositae	Amores
223.	Cosmos pringlei Robinson & Fernald	Compositae	Bavisa; Mata Gusano
224.	Coursetia glandulosa A. Gray	Leguminosae	Samán

BOTANICAL NAME		FAMILY	SPANISH NAME
225.	Coutarea sp. (see Hintonia)		
226.	Cowania plicata D. Don	Rosaceae	Alejandria
227.	Cowania sp.	Rosaceae	Romero Cedro
228.	Crataegus mexicana Moc. & Sessé	Rosaceae	Tejocote
229.	Crescentia alata H.B.K.	Bignoniaceae	Cuautecomate; Guaje Cirial
230.	Croton californicus Muell. Arg.	Euphorbiaceae	
231.	Croton corymbulosus Engelm. in Wheeler	Euphorbiaceae	Yerba del Gato
232.	Croton monanthogynus Michx.	Euphorbiaceae	Encinilla
233.	Croton niveus Jacq. ?	Euphorbiaceae	Verablanca
234.	Croton texensis (Klotzsch) Muell. Arg.	Euphorbiaceae	Barbasco
235.	Croton sp.	Euphorbiaceae	Majahui; Barbo; Yerba de Zorrillo
236.	Cucurbita digitata A. Gray	Cucurbitaceae	Calabasilla
237.	Cucurbita ficifolia Bouché	Cucurbitaceae	
238.	Cucurbita foetidissima H.B.K.	Cucurbitaceae	Calabazilla; Chilicoyote
239.	Cucurbita moschata Duch.	Cucurbitaceae	Calabasa
240.	Cuminum cyminum L. C. odorum Salisb.	Umbelliferae	Comino
241.	Cunila longiflora A. Gray	Labiatae	Poléo
242.	Cuphea aequipetala Cav.	Lythraceae	Yerba del Cancer
243.	Cupressus arizonica Greene	Pinaceae	
244.	Cupressus benthamii Endl.	Pinaceae	Cedro
245.	Cuscuta curta (Engelm.) Rydb.	Convolvulaceae	Cuscuta;Yerba Mala; Yerba sin Raiz

BOTANICAL NAME	FAMILY	SPANISH NAME
246. Cydonia see Pyrus		
247. Cymbopogon citratus (DC.) Stapf.	Gramineae	Zacate de Limon
248. Cymopterus purpureus S. Wats. Aulospermum purpureum (S. Wats.) Coult. & Rose	Umbelliferae	Chimaja
249. Dalea formosa Torr.	Leguminosae	Yerba de Alonso Garcia
250. Dalea polygonoides A. Gray	Leguminosae	
251. Dalea sp.	Leguminosae	Yerba de la Pulga; Ramon; Javonsillo or Jaronsillo
252. Dasylirion durangense Trel.	Liliaceae	Palmilla; Palma; Sotol
253. Dasylirion simplex Trel.	Liliaceae	Sotol
254. Dasylirion wheeleri S. Wats.	Liliaceae	Palmilla; Palma; Sotol
255. Datura candida Safford	Solanaceae	Florefundia; Florepondia; Bomba
256. Datura meteloides DC. ex Dunal	Solanaceae	Toloache; Tolache; Tolachi
257. Datura stramonium L.	Solanaceae	Toloache
258. Datura sp.	Solanaceae	Toloache; Estramonio
259. Daucus carota L.	Umbelliferae	Zanahoria
260. Descurainia pinnata (Walt.) Britton	Cruciferae	Pamita
261. Descurainia pinnata (Walt.) Britton ssp. meziessi (DC.) Detling Sophia pinnata (Walt.) Britton	Cruciferae	Pamita

BOTANICAL NAME	FAMILY	SPANISH NAME
262. *Dichondra argentea* Willd.	Convolvulaceae	Orejuela de Raton; Oreja de Raton; Golondrina
263. *Dichondra repens* Forst.	Convolvulaceae	
264. *Distichlis spicata* (L.) Greene	Gramineae	Yerba del Burro
265. *Dodonaea* sp.	Sapindaceae	Jarilla
266. *Drymaria gracilis* Cham. & Schlecht.	Caryophyllaceae	Yerba del Tomor
267. *Dryopteris normalis* C. Chr.	Polypodiaceae	
268. *Dryopteris pilosa* C. Chr.	Polypodiaceae	
269. *Dyschoriste decumbens* (Gray) Ktze.	Acanthaceae	Yerba de la Vivora
270. *Dyschoriste linearis* (Torr. & Gray) Ktze.	Acanthaceae	Yerba Vivora
271. *Dyssodia acerosa* DC.	Compositae	Yerba del Arriero
272. *Dyssodia papposa* (Vent.) Hitchc.	Compositae	Pagué
273. *Dyssodia pentachaeta* (DC.) Robinson	Compositae	Limoncillo
274. *Dyssodia setifolia* (Lag.) Robinson	Dompositae	Parralena; Parraleña
275. *Echeveria simulans* Rose	Crassulaceae	Yedra grande; Yedra del Monte
276. *Echinocereus paucispinus* Rümpler	Cactaceae	Pitajaya
277. *Echinocystis lobata* Torr. & Gray	Cucurbitaceae	Estrella del Norte
278. *Elaphrium pubescens* Schlecht. *Bursera pubescens* Standl.	Burseraceae	Zarzafras

BOTANICAL NAME	FAMILY	SPANISH NAME
279. Elytraria imbricata (Vahl.) Pers.	Acanthaceae	Cordoncillo
280. Encelia farinosa A. Gray in Emory	Compositae	Incienso; Yerba del Vaso; Palo Blanco; Yerba Ceniza
281. Enterolobium cyclocarpum (Jacq.) Griseb.	Leguminosae	Huinecastle
282. Ephedra antisyphilitica Meyer	Ephedraceae	Popotillo
283. Ephedra aspera Engelm.	Ephedraceae	Grangrene; Itamo Rial
284. Ephedra californica S. Wats.	Ephedraceae	Cañutillo
285. Ephedra torreyana S. Wats	Ephedraceae	Cañutillo del Campo; Caña-tilla; Popo-tillo; Tepo-pote
286. Equisetum arvense L. ?	Equisetaceae	Cañutillo
287. Equisetum hyemale L.	Equisetaceae	Cola de Caballo; Cañutillo del Llano
288. Equisetum laevigatum A. Br.	Equisetaceae	Cola de Caballo
289. Equisetum sp.	Equisetaceae	Carisillo; Cañolilla
290. Erigeron canadensis L.	Compositae	Pazotillo
291. Erigeron flagellaris A. Gray	Compositae	Zarzilla
292. Eriodictyon agustifolium Nutt.	Hydrophyllaceae	Yerba Santa
293. Eriodictyon crassifolium Benth.	Hydrophyllaceae	Yerba Santa

BOTANICAL NAME	FAMILY	SPANISH NAME
294. Eriogonum atrorubens Engelm.	Polygonaceae	Yerba Colorado
295. Eriogonum fasciculatum Benth.	Polygonaceae	
296. Eriogonum racemosum Nutt.	Polygonaceae	Colita de Rata; Colita de Raton
297. Eriogonum tenellum Torr.	Polygonaceae	Chuchaca
298. Eriogonum sp.	Polygonaceae	
299. Eriosema grandiflorum (Schlecht. & Cham.) Seem.	Leguminosae	Guayabillo
300. Erodium cicutarium (L.) L'Hér.	Geraniaceae	Yerba de Chuparrosa; Alfilerillo
301. Eruca sativa Mill. Brassica eruca L.	Cruciferae	Saramago
302. Eryngium carlinae Délar.	Umbelliferae	Yerba del Sapo
303. Eryngium hemsleyanum Wolff.	Umbelliferae	Yerba del Sapo
304. Eryngium rosei Hemsl.	Umbelliferae	
305. Eryngium wrightii A. Gray	Umbelliferae	Yerba del Sapo
306. Eryngium sp.	Umbelliferae	Yerba del Sapo
307. Erysimum capitatum (Dougl.) Greene E. elatum Nutt.	Cruciferae	Yerba del Apache
308. Erythrina flabelliformis Kearney	Leguminosae	Colorín; Chilicote; Chilocote; Frijolillo
309. Erythrina sp.	Leguminosae	
310. Eucalyptus sp.	Mirtaceae	Eucalita

BOTANICAL NAME	FAMILY	SPANISH NAME
311. *Eupatorium collinum* DC.	Compositae	Yerba de Angel
312. *Eupatorium deltoideum* Jacq.	Compositae	
313. *Eupatorium herbaceum* (A. Gray) Greene *E. arizonicum* (A. Gray) Greene	Compositae	Mata
314. *Eupatorium subintergrum* (Greene) Robinson	Compositae	Mula; de la Mula
315. *Eupatorium* sp.	Compositae	Peston
316. *Euphorbia albo-marginata* Torr. & Gray	Euphorbiaceae	Orejuela de Raton
317. *Euphorbia antisyphilitica* Zucc.	Euphorbiaceae	Candelilla
318. *Euphorbia heterophylla* L.	Euphorbiaceae	
319. *Euphorbia maculata* L.	Euphorbiaceae	Yerba de la Golondrina
320. *Euphorbia melanadenia* Torr.	Euphorbiaceae	Golondrina
321. *Euphorbia serpyllifolia* Pers.	Euphorbiaceae	Yerba de la Golondrina
322. *Euphorbia* sp.	Euphorbiaceae	Hierba de la Golondrina; Golondrina; Yerba de Coyote
323. *Exogonium bracteatum* (Cav.) Choisy	Convolvulaceae	Jícama
324. *Eysenhardtia polystachya* (Ortega) Sarg.	Leguminosae	Bura Dulce; Palo Azul
325. *Fallugia paradoxa* (D. Don) Endl.	Rosaceae	Poñil
326. *Ferocactus wislizenii* (Engelm.) Britt. & Rose	Cactaceae	Viznaga
327. *Ferocactus* sp.	Cactaceae	Biznaga

BOTANICAL NAME	FAMILY	SPANISH NAME
328. Ficus carica L.	Moraceae	Egara; Higos
329. Ficus cotinifolia H.B.K.	Moraceae	
330. Ficus petiolaris H.B.K.	Moraceae	Tescalama
331. Ficus radulina S. Wats.	Moraceae	Higuera
332. Fimbristylis sp.	Cyperaceae	
333. Flourensia cernua DC.	Compositae	Hojasen; Ojase
334. Foeniculum vulgare Mill.	Umbelliferae	Hinojo; Te de Hinojo
335. Fouquieria fasciculata (Roem. & Schult.) Nash	Fouquieriaceae	Torote; Ocotillo
336. Franseria acanthicarpa (Hook.) Coville	Compositae	Yerba del Sapo; Rosetilla; Estafiate
337. Franseria ambrosioides Cav.	Compositae	Chicura
338. Franseria confertiflora (DC.) Rydb. F. tenuifolia Harv. & Gray	Compositae	Yerba del Sapo
339. Franseria sp.	Compositae	Chicura; Yerba del Sapo
340. Frasera see Swertia		
341. Fraxinus sp.	Oleaceae	Fresno
342. Gaillardia nervosa Rydb.	Compositae	Arnica
343. Gaillardia pinnatifida Torr.	Compositae	Coronilla; Yerba del Sol
344. Galium sp.	Rubiaceae	Yerba del Coyote
345. Galpinsia hartwegii (Benth.) Britton	Onagraceae	Amapola
346. Garrya veatchii Kell.	Garryaceae	

BOTANICAL NAME	FAMILY	SPANISH NAME
347. *Gaura coccinea* Pursh *Goura coccinea* Nutt. in Fraser	Onagraceae	Yerba del Golpe; Yerba de la Virgen
348. *Gaura sinuata* Nutt. ex Ser.	Onagraceae	Yerba del Golpe
349. *Geranium caespitosum* James *G. atropurpureum* Heller	Geraniaceae	Patita de Leon
350. *Geranium mexicanum* H.B.K.	Geraniaceae	Pata de Leon
351. *Gilia* see *Ipomopsis*		
352. *Glycyrrhiza lepidota* (Nutt.) Pursh	Leguminosae	Amolillo; Raiz del Desierto
353. *Gnaphalium canescens* DC.	Compositae	Gordolobo
354. *Gnaphalium macounii* Greene	Compositae	Manzanilla del Rio; Gordolobo
355. *Gnaphalium semiamplexicaule* DC.	Compositae	Calampacate; Gordolobo
356. *Gnaphalium wrightii* A. Gray	Compositae	Manzanilla del Rio
357. *Gnaphalium* sp.	Compositae	Manzanilla del Rio; Gordolobo; Lampaquate
358. *Grindelia aphanactis* Rydb.	Compositae	Yerba del Buey; Pega-pega
359. *Grindelia oxylepis* Greene	Compositae	Arnica
360. *Grindelia squarrosa* (Pursh) Dunal	Compositae	
361. *Guazuma ulmifolia* Lam.	Sterculiaceae	Guásima; Bolitas Quasima; Guaccimas
362. *Gutierrezia linoides* Greene	Compositae	Coyaye

BOTANICAL NAME	FAMILY	SPANISH NAME
363. Gutierrezia longifolia Greene	Compositae	Coyaye
364. Gutierrezia sarothrae (Pursh) Britt. & Rusby G. tenuis Greene	Compositae	Escoba de la Vibora; Yerba de la Vibora; Collalle; Rosita
365. Gutierrezia sp.	Compositae	Yerba de la Vibora
366. Gymnosperma corymbosum DC. Selloa glutinosa Spreng.	Compositae	Jarilla; Tatalencho
367. Haematoxylum brasiletto Karst.	Leguminosae	Brazîl
368. Haematoxylum campechianum L.	Leguminosae	Brazîl
369. Haplopappus laricifolius A. Gray	Compositae	Yerba del Pasmo
370. Haplopappus spinulosus (Pursh) DC.	Compositae	Yerba de la Quintana
371. Haplopappus spinulosus (Pursh) DC., var. turbinellus (Rydb.) Blake	Compositae	Arnica
372. Haplopappus venetus Blake, ssp. furfuraceus (Greene) Hall	Compositae	
373. Haplopappus sp.	Compositae	Yerba de la Vibora
374. Haplophyton sp.	Apocynaceae	Yerba de la Cucaracha
375. Hedeoma dentatum Torr.	Labiatae	Yerba del Catarro
376. Hedeoma nanum (Torr.) Greene	Labiatae	Poléo
377. Hedeoma oblongifolium (Gray) Heller	Labiatae	Poléo Chino
378. Hedeoma piperitum Benth.	Labiatae	Tabajillo

BOTANICAL NAME	FAMILY	SPANISH NAME
379. *Heimia salicifolia* Link	Lythraceae	Yerba Jonequil
380. *Helenium hoopesii* Gray	Compositae	Yerba del Lobo
381. *Helenium mexicanum* H.B.K.	Compositae	Hierba Cabezona
382. *Helianthemum glomeratum* Lag. ex DC.	Cistaceae	Sanguinaria; Juanita; Hierba de la Gallina
383. *Helianthus annuus* L.	Compositae	Añil; Mira Sol
384. *Helianthus ciliaris* DC.	Compositae	Yerba Parda
385. *Heliocereus speciosus* (Cav.) Britt. & Rose	Cactaceae	Cola de Gato
386. *Heliotropium greggii* Torr.	Boraginaceae	Damiana
387. *Heracleum lanatum* Michx.	Umbelliferae	Yerba del Oso
388. *Heterotheca* sp.	Compositae	Arnica
389. *Hibiscus syriacus* L. ?	Malvaceae	Flor Altea
390. *Hieracium fendleri* Sch. Bip.	Compositae	Oreja del Raton; Oreja del Gato
391. *Hieracium* sp.	Compositae	Lechuvilla
392. *Hilaria cenchroides* H.B.K.	Granineae	Sacate Chino
393. *Hintonia latiflora* (DC.) Bullock *Coutarea latiflora* Moc. & Sessé *C. pterosperma* (S. Wats.) Standl.	Rubiaceae	Copalquín
394. *Hoffmanseggia densiflora* Benth. ex A. Gray	Leguminosae	Wisachito; Camote de Raton
395. *Hordeum vulgare* L.	Gramineae	Sevada

BOTANICAL NAME	FAMILY	SPANISH NAME
396. Houstonia acerosa A. Gray ?	Rubiaceae	Angrelitas
397. Humulus americanus Nutt. H. lupulus L., var. neo-mexicanus A. Nels. & Ckll.	Moraceae	Zarza, Zarzaparilla
398. Hura crepitans L.	Euphorbiaceae	Tescalama
399. Hymenoxys richardsonii (Hook.) Cockerell, var. floribunda (Gray) K.F. Parker	Compositae	Pinhué; Pingué; Pinguay
400. Hypericum pratense Schlecht. & Cham.	Hypericaceae	Sangrinaria
401. Hyptis albida H.B.K.	Labiatae	
402. Hyptis emoryi Torr.	Labiatae	Chía
403. Illicium verum Hook.	Illiciaceae	Anís Estrella
404. Indigofera suffruticosa Mill.	Leguminosae	
405. Ipomoea mexicana A. Gray I. purpurea Lam.	Convolvulaceae	Carriuela
406. Ipomoea sp.	Convolvulaceae	Espanto Vaquero; Tumbo Vaqueros
407. Ipomopsis longiflora (Torr.) V. Grant Gilia longiflora (Torr.) G. Don	Polemiaceae	Lina
408. Iresine calea (Ibáñez) Standl.	Amaranthaceae	Carricillo
409. Iresine interrupta Benth.	Amaranthaceae	
410. Iris sp.	Iridaceae	Lirio
411. Jacobinia spicigera (Schlecht.) L.H. Bailey	Acanthaceae	Muicle
412. Jatropha cardiophylla (Torr.) Muell. Arg.	Euphorbiaceae	Sangre de Cristo; Sangre de Drago

BOTANICAL NAME	FAMILY	SPANISH NAME
413. Jatropha cuneata Wiggins & Rollins	Euphorbiaceae	Torote
414. Jatropha curcas L.	Euphorbiaceae	Sangre Grado
415. Jatropha macrorhiza Benth.	Euphorbiaceae	
416. Juglans major (Torr.) Heller	Juglandaceae	Nogal
417. Juglans sp.	Juglandaceae	Nogal; Hojas de Nogal; Nuez
418. Juliania adstringens (Schlecht.) Schiede ex Schlecht.	Julianiaceae	Cascara
419. Juniperus californica Carr.	Cupressaceae	Guata
420. Juniperus communis L. J. sibirica Burgsd.	Cupressaceae	Sabina Macho; Pino Macho
421. Juniperus monosperma (Engelm.) Sarg.	Cupressaceae	Almaciga de Sabina; Sabina; Rama de Sabina
422. Juniperus pachyphloea Torr.	Cupressaceae	
423. Juniperus scopulorum Sarg.	Cupressaceae	Cedro
424. Juniperus spp.	Cupressaceae	Bellota de Sabina Tascate; Cuipa de Sabina; Cedro Colorado
425. Kallstroemia californica (S. Wats.) Vail, var. brachystylis (Vail) Kearney & Peebles	Zygophyllaceae	Contrayerba
426. Karwinskia humboldtiana (Roem. & Schult.) Zucc.	Rhamnaceae	Margarita; Cacachila; Palo Apestosa

BOTANICAL NAME	FAMILY	SPANISH NAME
427. Krameria grayi Rose & Painter K. canescens A. Gray	Leguminosae	Chacate
428. Krameria pauciflora Rose	Leguminosae	Zarzaparilla; Sarsaparilla; Cloradia; Clameria
429. Krameria sp.	Leguminosae	Chacate
430. Laelia sp.	Orchidaceae	Flor de San Diego
431. Lantana involucrata L.	Verbenaceae	Peonia
432. Lantana sp.	Verbenaceae	Sonorita; Majorana
433. Larrea tridentata (DC.) Coville divaricata Cav.	Zygophyllaceae	Gobernadora; Guamis; Wame Gobernadora; Hediondilla; Goma de Señora; Hediodia
434. Lathyrus decaphyllus Pursh	Leguminosae	Patito del Campo; Patito del País
435. Lathyrus eucosmus Butters & St. John L. decaphyllus Pursh	Leguminosae	
436. Lathyrus vernus Bernh.	Leguminosae	Oreja del Gato
437. Lavandula spica Cav.	Labiatae	Aluzema
438. Lavandula sp.	Labiatae	Alucema
439. Lemaireocereus sp.	Cactaceae	Pitajaya
440. Lemna sp.	Lemnaceae	Lentejilla; Lentejilla de Agua
441. Lepachys see Ratibida		
442. Lepechinia spicata Willd.	Labiatae	Betónica
443. Lepidium densiflorum Schrad. ?	Cruciferae	Lantejilla

BOTANICAL NAME	FAMILY	SPANISH NAME
444. *Lepidium virginicum* L., var. *pubescens* (Greene) C.L. Hitchcock	Cruciferae	Tapona
445. *Lepidium montanum* Nutt., var. *alyssoides* (A. Gray) M.E. Jones *L. alyssoides* A. Gray	Cruciferae	Mostacilla
446. *Lepidium virginicum* L.	Cruciferae	Lentajilla
447. *Leptodactylon* sp.	Polemoniaceae	Yerba del Coyote
448. *Leucaena* sp.	Leguminosae	Tepahuaje
449. *Leucophyllum laevigatum* Standl.	Scrophulariaceae	Seniso
450. *Leucophyllum zygophyllum* I.M. Johnst.	Scrophulariaceae	Cenizo
451. *Liatris* sp.	Compositae	Flor de Cachana
452. *Ligusticum porteri* Coult. & Rose	Umbelliferae	Osha; Chu-Chufate; Chuchupate
453. *Linum lewisii* Pursh	Linaceae	Linasa
454. *Lippia berlandieri* Schauer	Verbenaceae	Oregano
455. *Lippia dulcis* Trevir.	Verbenaceae	Yerba Dulce
456. *Lippia palmeri* S. Wats.	Verbenaceae	Oregano
457. *Lippia triphylla* (L'Hér.) Ktze.	Verbenaceae	Cedrón; Cedrón de Castilla
458. *Lippia* sp.	Verbenaceae	Yerba de la Mula
459. *Litsea glaucescens* H.B.K.	Lauraceae	Laurel
460. *Litsea pringlei* Bartlett	Lauraceae	Laurel
461. *Lobelia laxiflora* H.B.K.	Lobeliaceae	Guadalupe

BOTANICAL NAME	FAMILY	SPANISH NAME
462. *Loeselia coerulea* (Cav.) G. Don	Polemoniaceae	Guachichiligo
463. *Loeselia mexicana* (Lam.) Brand *L. coccinea* (Cav.) G. Don *L. coccinea* "Brand"	Polemoniaceae	Espinoncillo; Guachichile; Huichichili
464. *Loeselia* sp.	Polemoniaceae	Hinseseli; Guachichile; Espanita ?
465. *Lonicera subspicata* Hook. & Arn., var. *johnstonii* Keck	Caprifoliaceae	Moronel
466. *Lophophora williamsii* (Lem.) Coulter	Cactaceae	Peyote
467. *Lupinus aduncus* Greene	Leguminosae	Garbancillo
468. *Lycium pallidum* Miers	Solanaceae	Chico; Tomatillo
469. *Lycium schaffneri* A. Gray	Solanaceae	Pico Pajaro
470. *Lycium* sp.	Solanaceae	Pinole
471. *Lycopersicon esculentum* Mill.	Solanaceae	Jitomate
472. *Lycurus phleoides* H.B.K.	Gramineae	Sacate Cola Sorra
473. *Lygodesmia juncea* (Pursh) D. Don	Compositae	Chiquete de Embarañada; Chicote Enbarrañada
474. *Lysiloma watsonii* Rose	Leguminosae	Tepeguaje
475. *Macrosiphonia hypoleuca* (Benth.) Muell. Arg.	Apocynaceae	Rosa de San Pedro
476. *Macrosiphonia lanuginosa* (Mart. & Gal.) Hemsl.	Apocynaceae	Flor de San Juan
477. *Magnolia schiedeana* Schlecht.	Magnoliaceae	
478. *Magnolia* sp.	Magnoliaceae	Corpus

BOTANICAL NAME	FAMILY	SPANISH NAME
479. *Malva crispa* L.	Malvaceae	Malva de Castilla
480. *Malva parviflora* L.	Malvaceae	Malvas; Malva; Malva del Campo
481. *Malva rotundifolia* L.	Malvaceae	Malva
482. *Malvaviscus aboreus* Cav.	Malvaceae	Malva
483. *Malvaviscus conzattii* Greenm.	Malvaceae	Flor de Molenillo
484. *Malvaviscus* sp.	Malvaceae	Monasillo; Manzanilla
485. *Mammea americana* L.	Guttiferae	Hueso de Mamey
486. *Mammillaria heyderi* Mühlenpf.	Cactaceae	Biznago
487. *Marrubium vulgare* L.	Labiatae	Marrubio; Mastrânzo; Concha
488. *Martynia* see *Proboscidea*		
489. *Mascagnia macroptera* (Moc. & Sessé) Niedenzu	Loganiaceae	
490. *Matelea* sp.	Asclepiadaceae	
491. *Matricaria chamomilla* L. *M. courrantiana* DC.	Compositae	Manzanilla; Manzanilla de Castilla;
492. *Matricaria matricarioides* (Less.) Porter	Compositae	Manzanilla
493. *Matricaria* sp.	Compositae	Manzanilla
494. *Medicago sativa* L.	Leguminosae	Alfalfa
495. *Melilotus alba* Desr.	Leguminosae	Alfalfón
496. *Melilotus indica* (L.) All.	Leguminosae	Trébol
497. *Menodora coulteri* A. Gray	Oleaceae	San Nicolas

BOTANICAL NAME	FAMILY	SPANISH NAME
498. *Mentha arvensis* L. *M. canadensis* L.	Labiatae	Polêo del Paris; Poléo Grande; Yerba Buena; Polêo
499. *Mentha spicata* L.	Labiatae	Yerba Buena
500. *Mentha* sp.	Labiatae	Yerba Buena; Poléo
501. *Mentzelia hispida* Willd.	Loasaceae	Pega Ropa
502. *Mentzelia multiflora* (Nutt.) A. Gray	Loasaceae	Pegapega
503. *Mikania guaco* Humb. & Bompl.	Compositae	Guaco
504. *Milla biflora* Cav.	Liliaceae	Carcoma; Estrella
505. *Mimosa biuncifera* Benth.	Leguminosae	Garavàtillo
506. *Mimulus guttatus* DC.	Scrophulariaceae	Berro; Lantén Cimarrón
507. *Mirabilis froebelii* Greene, var. *glabrata* (Standl.) Jepson	Nyctaginaceae	Yerba del Indio
508. *Mirabilis multiflora* (Torr.) A. Gray *Quamoclidion multiflorum* Torr.	Nyctaginaceae	Maravilla
509. *Monarda menthifolia* Graham	Labiatae	Orégano; Orégano de la Sierra
510. *Monarda pectinata* Nutt.	Labiatae	Orégano del Campo
511. *Mucuna* sp.	Leguminosae	Ojo de Venado
512. *Muhlenbergia dumosa* Scribn.	Gramineae	Otatillo
513. *Muhlenbergia emersleyi* Vasey	Gramineae	Cola de Ratón
514. *Muhlenbergia monticola* Buckl.	Gramineae	Zacate Liso

BOTANICAL NAME		FAMILY	SPANISH NAME
515.	Muhlenbergia porteri Scribn. ex Beal	Gramineae	
516.	Nama hispidum A. Gray	Hydrophyllaceae	Bentosidad
517.	Nama palmeri A. Gray	Hydrophyllaceae	Bentosidad
518.	Nama undulatum H.B.K.	Hydrophyllaceae	Ventosidad; Ventocidad
519.	Nepeta sp.	Labiatae	Toronjil de China
520.	Nerium oleander L.	Apocynaceae	Laurel
521.	Nicotiana attenuata Torr.	Solanaceae	Tabaco Coyote; Punche
522.	Nicotiana glauca Graham	Solanaceae	
523.	Nicotiana rustica L.	Solanaceae	Punche
524.	Nicotiana tabacum L.	Solanaceae	Tabaco Cimarrón
525.	Nicotiana trigonophylla Dunal	Solanaceae	Tobaca Loco
526.	Nicotiana sp.	Solanaceae	Punche Macuchi
527.	Nolina durangensis Trel.	Liliaceae	Palmilla
528.	Nolina matapensis Wiggins	Liliaceae	Palmilla
529.	Nolina microcarpa S. Wats.	Liliaceae	Sacahuista
530.	Nolina sp.	Liliaceae	Nolina
531.	Notholaena candida (Mort. & Gal.) Hook.	Polypodiaceae	Calaguala
532.	Notholaena sinuata (Lag.) Kaulf.	Polypodiaceae	Calahua del Indio; Calaguala
533.	Notholaena sinuata (Lag.) Kaulf., var. integerrima Hook.	Polypodiaceae	Canahuala

BOTANICAL NAME	FAMILY	SPANISH NAME
534. Nymphaea (probably ampla DC.)	Nymphaeaceae	Flor de la Paz
535. Ocimum basilicum L.	Labiatae	Alvacar; Albahaca
536. Ocimum micranthum Willd.	Labiatae	Albahaca
537. Oenothera greggii A. Gray, var. pringelei Munz	Onagraceae	Amapola
538. Oenothera laciniata Hill	Onagraceae	Amapola
539. Oenothera mexicana Spach	Onagraceae	Yerba del Golpe
540. Oenothera rosea Ait.	Onagraceae	Amapola; Yerba del Golpe
541. Oenothera runcinata (Engelm.) Munz Anogra runcinata (Engelm.) Woot. & Standl.	Onagraceae	Flor de San Juan
542. Oenothera triloba Nutt.	Onagraceae	Amapola
543. Opuntia imbricata (Haw.) DC. O. arborescens Engelm.	Cactaceae	Entraña; Pitajaya; Velas de Coyote
544. Opuntia leptocaulis DC.	Cactaceae	Garrambullo; Tasajilla
545. Opuntia parryi Engelm.	Cactaceae	Cholla
546. Opuntia sp.	Cactaceae	Nopal
547. Oryza sativa L.	Gramineae	Arroz
548. Oxalis albicans H.B.K.	Oxalidaceae	Socoyolle; Agrito
549. Oxalis leonis Knuth	Oxalidaceae	Agrito
550. Oxalis violacea L.	Oxalidaceae	Socoyol; Chocoyle; Jocoyol
551. Oxytropis lambertii Pursh	Leguminosae	Frijollillo

BOTANICAL NAME	FAMILY	SPANISH NAME
552. *Pachycereus pecten-arboriginum* (Engelm.) Britt. & Rose	Cactaceae	Cardón; Hecho; Pitajaya
553. *Paeonia* sp.	Ranunculaceae	Peonía
554. *Panicum obtusum* H.B.K.	Gramineae	Sacate Masarca
555. *Papaver rhoeas* L.	Papaveraceae	
556. *Parietaria pensylvanica* Muhl.	Urticaceae	Tripa de Judas
557. *Parkinsonia aculeata* L.	Leguminosae	Mezquite Extranjero
558. *Parmelia reticulata* Tayl.	Parmeliaceae	Flor de Piedra
559. *Parthenium argentatum* A. Gray in Torr.	Compositae	Guayale
560. *Parthenium confertum* A. Gray, var. *lyratum* A. Gray *P. lyratum* (A. Gray) A. Gray	Compositae	Altimisa
561. *Parthenium incanum* H.B.K.	Compositae	Mariola
562. *Pectis angustifolia* Torr.	Compositae	Limoncillo
563. *Pectis stenophylla* A. Gray	Compositae	
564. *Pedilanthus pavonis* (Klotzsch & Garcke) Boiss. in DC.	Euphorbiaceae	Yerba Candelilla
565. *Pedilanthus* sp. ?	Euphorbiaceae	
566. *Pelargonium graveoleus* L'Hér.	Geraniaceae	Geranio
567. *Pellaea cordata* (Cav.) Sm.	Polypodiaceae	Itamo real; Agritos
568. *Peniocereus* sp.	Cactaceae	Reina de la Noche
569. *Penstemon barbatus* (Cav.) Roth, ssp. *torreyi* (Benth.) Keck *P. torreyi* Benth.	Scrophulariaceae	Varas de San José; Varitas de San José

BOTANICAL NAME	FAMILY	SPANISH NAME
570. *Penstemon centranthifolius* Benth.	Scrophulariaceae	
571. *Penstemon* sp.	Scrophulariaceae	Varitas de San José
572. *Perezia nana* A. Gray	Compositae	Pichichagua
573. *Perezia runcinata* Lag.	Compositae	Piania
574. *Pericome caudata* A. Gray	Compositae	Yerba del Chivato
575. *Persea americana* Mill.	Laureaceae	Aguacate; Laurelillo
576. *Peteria* sp.	Leguminosae	Camote de Monte
577. *Petroselinum* see *Carum*		
578. *Peucephyllum* sp.	Compositae	
579. *Peumus boldus* Mol.	Monimiaceae	Boldo
580. *Phaseolus metcalfei* Woot. & Standl.	Leguminosae	Corcomeca; Frijolillo
581. *Phaseolus vulgaris* L.	Leguminosae	Frijoles
582. *Phlox nana* Nutt.	Polemoniaceae	Rosita Morada
583. *Phoradendron juniperinum* Engelm.	Loranthaceae	Bellota de Sabina
584. *Phragmites communis* Trin.	Gramineae	Carrizo
585. *Phragmites* sp.	Gramineae	Carrizo
586. *Physalis neomexicana* Rydb.	Solanaceae	Tomate del Campo; Tomate
587. *Physalis sordida* Fernald	Solanaceae	Tomate de Campo
588. *Physalis* sp.	Solanaceae	Tomatilla; Costomate
589. *Picramnia* sp.	Simaroubaceae	Colpaquín

BOTANICAL NAME	FAMILY	SPANISH NAME
590. <u>Picrasma</u> <u>excelsa</u> Planch. in Hook.	Simaroubaceae	Quasia
591. <u>Pimpinella</u> <u>anisum</u> L.	Umbelliferae	Anís; anís Chico
592. <u>Pinaropappus</u> <u>roseus</u> (Less.) Less.	Compositae	Ixpule
593. <u>Pinus</u> <u>arizonica</u> Engelm.	Pinaceae	
594. <u>Pinus</u> <u>ayacahuite</u> K.Ehrenb.	Pinaceae	Pino
595. <u>Pinus</u> <u>edulis</u> Engelm.	Pinaceae	Piñon
596. <u>Pinus</u> <u>engelmanni</u> Carr. <u>P.</u> <u>ponderosa</u> Dougl.	Pinaceae	
597. <u>Pinus</u> <u>leiophylla</u> Schlecht. & Cham.	Pinaceae	
598. <u>Pinus</u> <u>ponderosa</u> Lawson <u>P.</u> <u>brachyptera</u> Engelm.	Pinaceae	Pino Real Colorado
599. <u>Pinus</u> <u>ponderosa</u> Lawson, var. <u>scopulorum</u> Engelm.	Pinaceae	Pinavete
600. <u>Pinus</u> <u>reflexa</u> Engelm.	Pinaceae	
601. <u>Pinus</u> sp.	Pinaceae	Trementina; Ocote; Palo de Ocote
602. <u>Piper</u> <u>nigrum</u> L.	Piperaceae	Pimienta
603. <u>Piper</u> sp.	Piperaceae	Kokolmika
604. <u>Piqueria</u> <u>trinervia</u> Cav.	Compositae	Harta Reina; Alta Reina Tabardillo
605. <u>Pisonia</u> <u>capitata</u> (S. Wats.) Standl.	Nyctaginaceae	Bainora Prieto
606. <u>Pisum</u> <u>satium</u> L.	Leguminosae	Alberjón
607. <u>Pithecoctenium</u> <u>echinatum</u> Schlecht.	Bignoniaceae	Gueso de Mamell
608. <u>Pithecoctenium</u> sp.	Bignoniaceae	Bejuco de Huico

BOTANICAL NAME	FAMILY	SPANISH NAME
609. *Pithecellobium dulce* (Roxb.) Benth.	Mimosaceae	Guamúchil
610. *Plantago major* L.	Plantaginaceae	Lantén; Lantena; Semilla de Llantén; Venado
611. *Plantago* sp.	Plantaginaceae	Lantên
612. *Platanus wrightii* S. Wats.	Platanaceae	Aliso
613. *Pluchea sericea* (Nutt.) Coville	Compositae	Cachanilla
614. *Plumbago scandens* L.	Plumbaginaceae	
615. *Plumeria acutifolia* Poir.	Apocynaceae	
616. *Poinsettia radicans* (Benth.) Klotzsch & Garcke	Euphorbiaceae	A contra yerba
617. *Polianthes tuberosa* L.	Amaryllidaceae	Azucena
618. *Polygonum aviculare* L.	Polygonaceae	Lengua de Pajare
619. *Polygonum hydropiper* L.	Polygonaceae	Chilillo
620. *Polygonum hydropiperoides* Michx.	Polygonaceae	Chilillo
621. *Polygonum pensylvanicum* L.	Polygonaceae	Yerba del Pescado
622. *Polypodium aureum* L. ?	Polypodiaceae	
623. *Polypodium aviculare* L.	Polypodiaceae	
624. *Polypodium lanceolatum* L.	Polypodiaceae	Lengua de Cervo
625. *Populus angustifolia* James in Long	Salicaceae	Álamo Sauco
626. *Populus fremontii* S. Wats.	Salicaceae	Álamo
627. *Populus tremuloides* Michx.	Salicaceae	Alamillo; Álamo

BOTANICAL NAME		FAMILY	SPANISH NAME
628.	Populus wislizenii (S.Wats.) Sarg.	Salicaceae	Álamo de Hoja Redonda
629.	Populus sp.	Salicaceae	Cortesa de Álamo Blanco
630.	Porophyllum filifolium A. Gray not DC. P. filiforme Rydb.	Compositae	Benna dia; Yerba del Venado
631.	Porophyllum gracile Benth.	Compositae	Yerba del Venado
632.	Portulaca oleracea L.	Portulacaceae	Verdolaga
633.	Potentilla thurberi A.Gray ex Lehm.	Rosaceae	Clameria; Yerba Colorada; Fresa Cimarrona
634.	Potentilla sp. cf. exsul Standl.	Rosaceae	Fresa
635.	Proboscidea fragrans (Lindl.) Dcne. Martynia fragrans Lindl.	Martyniaceae	Gàrumbullo
636.	Prosopis chilensis (Mol.) Stuntz	Leguminosae	Corteza de Mezquite; Mesquite
637.	Prosopis juliflora Benth., var. torreyana L. Benson	Leguminosae	Mesquite
638.	Prosopis pubescens Benth. Strombocarpa pubescens (Benth.) A. Gray	Leguminosae	Tornillo
639.	Prunus armeniaca L.	Rosaceae	Amarrio; Hueso de Albaricoque
640.	Prunus brachybotrya Zucc.	Rosaceae	
641.	Prunus capuli Cav.	Rosaceae	Capulîn Pequeño; Corteza de Capulîn
642.	Prunus cerasus L.	Rosaceae	Hueso de Cereza

BOTANICAL NAME	FAMILY	SPANISH NAME
643. Prunus ilicifolia (Nutt.) Walp.	Rosaceae	Islaya
644. Prunus persica (L.) Batsch.	Rosaceae	Durazno
645. Prunus virginiana L., var. melanocarpa (A. Nels.) Sarg. P. melanocarpa (A. Nels.) Rydb.	Rosaceae	Capulín
646. Pseudotsuga taxifolia (Poir.) Britton P. mucronata	Pinaceae	Pino Real
647. Psidium guajava L.	Myrtaceae	Guayaba
648. Psoralea pentaphylla L.	Leguminosae	Contrayerba
649. Psoralea sp.	Leguminosae	Contra Yerba
650. Ptelea trifoliata L.	Rutaceae	
651. Pterocarpus acapulcensis Rose	Leguminosae	Drago
652. Punica granatum L.	Punicaceae	Granada
653. Purshia tridentata DC.	Rosaceae	
654. Pyrus cydonia L. Cydonia oblonga Mill.	Rosaceae	Capulîn
655. Quamoclidion see Mirabilis		
656. Quercus arizonica Sarg.	Fagaceae	
657. Quercus chihuahuensis Trel.	Fagaceae	
658. Quercus emoryi Torr.	Fagaceae	Bellota
659. Quercus endlichiana Trel.	Fagaceae	Popuisoli
660. Quercus gambelii Nutt.	Fagaceae	Encino; Encino de la Hoja Ancha
661. Quercus undulata Torr. Q. fendleri Liebm.	Fagaceae	Encinillo
662. Quercus viminea Trel.	Fagaceae	

BOTANICAL NAME	FAMILY	SPANISH NAME
663. Quercus sp.	Fagaceae	Encina
664. Randia echinocarpa Moc. & Sessé	Rubiaceae	Papache
665. Randia laevigata Standl.	Rubiaceae	
666. Randia watsonii Robinson	Rubiaceae	Papache Grande
667. Ranunculus sp.	Ranunculaceae	Diente; Muela; Remedio
668. Ratibida mexicana (S.Wats.) W.M. Sharp	Compositae	
669. Ratibida tagetes (James) Barnhart Lepachys tagetes A. Gray	Compositae	Yerba de la Tusa; Embarrañda
670. Ratibida tagetes (James) Barnhart Rudbeckia tagetes James	Compositae	Dormilón
671. Rhamnus californica Esch.	Rhamnaceae	Cáscara Sagrada
672. Rhus microphylla Engelm.	Anacardiaceae	Pico de Pajaro
673. Rhus ovata S. Wats.	Anacardiaceae	Mangle
674. Rhus radicans L. R. toxicodendron L.	Anacardiaceae	Yedra
675. Rhus trilobata Nutt.	Anacardiaceae	Lemita
676. Rhynchosia pyramidalis (Lam.) Urb.	Leguminosae	Ojo de Chanate; Chante Pusi
677. Ribes inebrians Lindl.	Saxifragaceae	Manzanita
678. Ribes neglectum Rose	Saxifragaceae	
679. Ricinus communis L.	Euphorbiaceae	Digerillo; Higuera; Higería; Higuerilla; Semillas Higeron

BOTANICAL NAME	FAMILY	SPANISH NAME
680. Robinia neomexicana A. Gray	Leguminosae	Uña de Gato
681. Rorippa nasturtium-aquaticum (L.) Schinz & Thell. Radicula nasturtium-aquaticum (L.) Britten & Rendle Nasturtium officinale R.Br.	Cruciferae	Berro
682. Rosa centifolia L.	Rosaceae	Rosa de Castillo
683. Rosa fendleri Crepín	Rosaceae	Rosa Cimarron; Rosa del Campo; Sencilla
684. Rosa sp.	Rosaceae	Rosa del Castillo; Rosa de Castilla
685. Rosmarinus officinalis L.	Labiatae	Romero
686. Rubus idaeus L., var. strigosus (Michx.) Maxim.	Rosaceae	Zarza Mora
687. Rudbeckia laciniata L.	Compositae	Dormilón
688. Rumex crispus L.	Polygonaceae	Yerba Colorado; Lengua de Vaca
689. Rumex hymenosepalus Torr.	Polygonaceae	Caña Agria; Canaigre; Canaigra
690. Rumex mexicanus Meisn.	Polygonaceae	Lengua de Vaca
691. Ruta chalepensis L.	Rutaceae	Ruda
692. Ruta graveolens L.	Rutaceae	Ruda
693. Ruta sp.	Rutaceae	Ruda
694. Sabal uresana Trel.	Palmae	Palma
695. Saccharum officinarum L.	Gramineae	Caña
696. Salix amygdaloides Anderss.	Salicaceae	

BOTANICAL NAME		FAMILY	SPANISH NAME
697.	Salix argophylla Nutt.	Salicaceae	Jara
698.	Salix exigua Nutt. (round-leafed variety)	Salicaceae	Jarita
699.	Salix mexicana Seemen	Salicaceae	Cocolmeca; Raiz de China
700.	Salvia apiana Jepson	Labiatae	Salvarial
701.	Salvia chamaedryoides Cav.	Labiatae	Mirto
702.	Salvia columbariae Benth.	Labiatae	Chîa
703.	Salvia hispanica L. or S. tiliaefolia Vahl.	Labiatae	Salvia
704.	Salvia mexicana L.	Labiatae	
705.	Salvia microphylla H.B.K.	Labiatae	Mirto
706.	Salvia pachyphylla Epl. ex Munz	Labiatae	Salvarial de la Sierra
707.	Salvia reflexa Hornem.	Labiatae	Chan; Chîa
708.	Salvia sp.	Labiatae	Mirto de Castilla
709.	Sambucus caerulea Raf.	Caprifoliaceae	Saúco
710.	Sambucus mexicana Presl	Caprifoliaceae	Sauco; Sauca; Flor de Sauz; Capulín Silvestre; Flor de Saugua; Flor Sauco
711.	Sanvitalia aberti A. Gray	Compositae	Yerba Fria
712.	Sanvitalia ocymoides DC.	Compositae	Flor de un Día
713.	Sanvitalia procumbens Lam.	Compositae	Ojo de Gallo
714.	Sapindus saponaria L., var. drummondii (Hook & Arn.) Benson	Sapindaceae	Jaboncillo
715.	Sapindus sp.	Sapindaceae	Palo Blanco

BOTANICAL NAME	FAMILY	SPANISH NAME
716. Sapium biloculare (S.Wats.) Pax in Engl.	Euphorbiaceae	Yerba de la Flecha
717. Saponaria officinalis L.	Caryophyllaceae	Clavelina; Clavellina
718. Saracha jaltomata Schlecht.	Solanaceae	Jaltomate
719. Sarcostemma cynanchoides Decne., ssp. hartwegii (Vail) R. Holm Funastrum heterophyllum (Engelm.) Standl.	Asclepiadaceae	Moradillo
720. Schinus molle L.	Anacardiaceae	Pirun; Pirul
721. Schrankia potosina (Britt. & Rose) Standl.	Leguminosae	Berguensa; Yerba de la Verguenza
722. Scirpus sp.	Cyperaceae	
723. Scoparia sp.	Scrophulariaceae	Yerba del Golpe
724. Scutellaria sp.	Labiatae	Albacar
725. Sebastiana pavoniana Muell. Arg.	Euphorbiaceae	
S. pringlei S. Wats.	Euphorbiaceae	Yerba de la Flecha
726. Sedum sp.	Crassulaceae	Siempreviva
727. Selaginella cuspidata Spring	Selaginellaceae	Chayotillo Flor de Peña
728. Selaginella sp.	Selaginellaceae	Flor de Peña Pescaditos del Cerro
729. Selloa see Gymnosperma		
730. Senecio sp. cf. actinella Greene	Compositae	Lechuguilla
731. Senecio filifolius Nutt.	Compositae	Yerba del Caballo
732. Senecio hartwegii Benth.	Compositae	

BOTANICAL NAME	FAMILY	SPANISH NAME
733. Senecio multicapitatus Greenm.	Compositae	Yerba del Caballo
734. Senecio salignus DC.	Compositae	Jarilla
735. Senecio sp.	Compositae	Lechuguilla; Lechuguilla de la Sierra
736. Serjania mexicana (L.) Willd.	Sapindaceae	Diente de Culebra; Guirote de Culebra; Diente de Vibora
737. Serjania triquetra Radlk.	Sapindaceae	Tres Costillas
738. Sesamum indicum L. S. orientale L.	Pedalineae	Ajonjoli
739. Sida cordifolia L.	Malvaceae	Malva
740. Sida hederacea (Dougl. ex Hook.) Torr. ex A. Gray	Malvaceae	Melonsilla
741. Sida procumbens Swartz	Malvaceae	Yerba del Buen Día
742. Sida rhombifolia L.	Malvaceae	Malva
743. Sitanion hystrix (Nutt.) J.G. Smith	Gramineae	Sacate Sevaidilla
744. Smilax cordifolia Humb. & Bonpl.	Liliaceae	Rais de China
745. Solanum diversifolium Schlecht.	Solanaceae	
746. Solanum elaeagnifolium Cav.	Solanaceae	Trompillo; Tomatillo del Campo; Tomatito Pelon; Tomatillo; Tomatito
747. Solanum fontanesianum Dunal	Solanaceae	Flor de Nacahuite

BOTANICAL NAME	FAMILY	SPANISH NAME
748. Solanum jamesii Torr.	Solanaceae	Papa Cimarrön
749. Solanum madrense Fernald	Solanaceae	Flor de Clamaclancle; Saca Manteca
750. Solanum nigrum L.	Solanaceae	Yerba Mora; Chichiquelite; Quelite; Yerba Nora; Tomatito
751. Solanum nodiflorum Jacq.	Solanaceae	Chichiquelite
752. Solanum pterocaulum Dunal	Solanaceae	Yerba Mora
753. Solanum rostratum Dunal	Solanaceae	Mala Mujer
754. Solanum tuberosum L.	Solanaceae	Papas
755. Solanum verbascifolium L.	Solanaceae	
756. Solidago canadensis L.	Compositae	Mariquilla
757. Sonchus arvensis L.	Compositae	Cerraja
758. Sonchus oleraceus L.	Compositae	Borraja
759. Sophia see Descurainia		
760. Sphaeralcea ambigua A. Gray	Malvaceae	
761. Sphaeralcea angustifolia (Cav.) G. Don, var. cuspidata A. Gray S. cuspidata (A. Gray) Britton	Malvaceae	Yerba del Negro; Yerba Negrito
762. Sphaeralcea angustifolia (Cav.) G. Don, var. lobata (Woot.) Kern. S. lobata	Malvaceae	Yerba del Negro
763. Sphaeralcea angustifolia "Spach"	Malvaceae	Yerba del Negro
764. Sphaeralcea fendleri A.Gray	Malvaceae	Yerba de la Negrita

BOTANICAL NAME	FAMILY	SPANISH NAME
765. Sphaeralcea hastatula A. Gray	Malvaceae	Yerba del Negrito; Yerba de Negro
766. Sphaeralcea sp.	Malvaceae	Mal de Ojos
767. Sporobolus wrightii Munro ex Scribn.	Granimeae	Sacatón
768. Stemmadenia palmeri Rose & Standl.	Gentianaceae	
769. Stevia micrantha Lag.	Compositae	
770. Stevia salicifolia Cav.	Compositae	
771. Stevia serrata Cav.	Compositae	
772. Stevia stenophylla A. Gray	Compositae	Yerba de la Virgen
773. Stevia sp.	Compositae	Hierba de la Mula
774. Stipa robusta (Vasey) Scribn. S. vaseyi Scribn.	Gramineae	Popotón; Scatón; Sacatón
775. Strombocarpa see Prosopis		
776. Struthanthus diversifolius (Benth.) Standl.	Bromeliaceae	Muérdago
777. Suaeda sp.	Chenopodiaceae	Quelite Salado
778. Swertia radiata (Kell.) Ktze. Frasera speciosa Hook.	Gentianaceae	Cebadilla; Cebadilla de la Sierra
779. Swietenia humilis Zucc.	Meliaceae	Flor de Venodillo
780. Tabebuia palmeri Rose	Bignoniaceae	
781. Tagetes erecta L.	Compositae	Flor de Muerto

BOTANICAL NAME	FAMILY	SPANISH NAME
782. Tagetes florida Sweet	Compositae	Pericón; Yerba Nis; Santa Maria; Operion
783. Tagetes jaliscensis Greenm.	Compositae	
784. Tagetes lucida Cav.	Compositae	Yerba Nil; Coronilla
785. Tagetes micrantha Cav.	Compositae	Anisillo
786. Tagetes sp.	Compositae	Cinco Yagay; Yerbanis
787. Talauma mexicana (DC.) G. Don	Magnoliaceae	Petales de Yolozochitl; Flor de Corazon
788. Tamarindus indica L.	Leguminosae	Tamarindo
789. Tanacetum vulgare L.	Compositae	Ponso; Tansê; Altamisa
790. Taonabo sp. (probably T. oocarpa Rose)	Ternstroemiaceae	Flor de Tilia de Estrella
791. Taraxacum officinale Weber in Wiggers	Compositae	Chicória
792. Taraxacum sp.	Compositae	Consuelda
793. Taxodium mucronatum Ten.	Pinaceae	Sabino
794. Tecoma stans (L.) H.B.K.	Bignoniaceae	Palo Amarillo
795. Tecoma sp.	Bignoniaceae	Retana; Retama
796. Tephrosia leiocarpa A.Gray	Leguminosae	
797. Tephrosia nicaraguensis Oerst.	Leguminosae	Yerba del Piojo
798. Ternstroemia pringlei Standl.	Ternstroemiaceae	Flor de Tilia

BOTANICAL NAME	FAMILY	SPANISH NAME
799. Thalictrum fendleri Engelm.	Ranunculaceae	Paloma Consulta; Ruda de la Sierra; Ruda Cimarrón
800. Thelesperma megapotamicum (Spreng) Ktze. T. gracile A. Gray T. longipes A. Gray	Compositae	Cota; Te Silvestre; Te; Te de los Navajos
801. Thelesperma trifidum (Lam.) Britton	Compositae	
802. Thevetia thevatioides (H. B.K.) K. Schum.	Apocynaceae	Codo de Fraile
803. Thryallis glauca (Cav.) Ktze.	Malpighiaceae	Ciruelo del Campo
804. Tilia sp.	Tiliaceae	Flor de Tilia; Trompa Roja
805. Tillandsia benthamiana (Beer) Baker	Bromeliaceae	
806. Tillandsia karwinskyana Schult.	Bromeliaceae	
807. Tillandsia recurvata L.	Bromeliaceae	Paschtle; Pastle de Mesquite
808. Tithonia fruticosa Canby & Rose	Compositae	
809. Tournefortia densiflora Mart. & Gal.	Boraginaceae	Yerba Rasposa
810. Tournefortia sp.	Boraginaceae	Yerba del Negro
811. Tragia nepetaefolia Cav.	Euphorbiaceae	Ortiguilla
812. Tragia ramosa Torr.	Euphorbiaceae	
813. Trichostema lanatum Benth.	Labiatae	
814. Trichostema parishii Vasey	Labiatae	Romero
815. Trifolium sp.	Leguminosae	Trebol

BOTANICAL NAME	FAMILY	SPANISH NAME
816. *Triticum* sp.	Gramineae	Trigo
817. *Trixis californica* Kell.	Compositae	Cachano
818. *Trixis* sp. cf. *radialis* (L.) Ktze.	Compositae	Yerba del Aire
819. *Turnera diffusa* Willd. *T. humifusa* (Presl) Endl. ex Walp.	Turneraceae	Damiana
820. *Turnera ulmifolia* L.	Turneraceae	
821. *Typha latifolia* L.	Typhaceae	Aguapá
822. *Ulmus lesueurii* Standl. or *U. mexicana* Planch. in DC.	Ulmaceae	Fruita Amarilla
823. *Urtica gracilis* Ait.	Urticaceae	Ortiguilla
824. *Usnea* sp.	Usneaceae	
825. *Valeriana* sp.	Valerianaceae	Raiz de Valeriana
826. *Verbascum thapsus* L.	Scrophulariaceae	Punchón; Tobaco Cimarrón; Candelaria; Gordolobo; Verbasco
827. *Verbena ambrosiaefolia* Rydb.	Verbenaceae	Moradilla
828. *Verbena carolina* L. ? *V. caroliniana* Willd.	Verbenaceae	Verbena
829. *Verbena ciliata* Benth.	Verbenaceae	Verbena
830. *Verbena elegans* H.B.K., var. *asperata* Perry	Verbenaceae	Verbena; Alfrombrillo
831. *Verbena macdougalii* Heller	Verbenaceae	Vervená; Dormilón
832. *Verbena polystachya* H.B.K.	Verbenaceae	Yerba de San José
833. *Verbena wrightii* A. Gray	Verbenaceae	Moradilla
834. *Verbesina encelioides* (Cav.) Benth.	Compositae	Añil del Muerto

BOTANICAL NAME	FAMILY	SPANISH NAME
835. Vicia faba L.	Leguminosae	Habas
836. Viguiera grammatoglossa DC.	Compositae	
837. Viguiera helianthoides H.B.K.	Compositae	Mirasol
838. Viola sp.	Violaceae	Violeta
839. Vitex mollis H.B.K.	Verbenaceae	Jari; Igual-amo
840. Vitis arizonica Engelm.	Vitaceae	Uva cimarrona; Envolver
841. Waltheria americana L.	Sterculiaceae	Yerba del Angel; Yerba del Pasmo
842. Wedeliella glabra (Choisy) Cockerell ?	Nyctaginaceae	Yerba de la Hormiga; Tê de la Hormiga
843. Wigandia kunthii Choisy	Hydrophyllaceae	Flor de Chicascle
844. Willardia mexicana (S.Wats.) Rose	Leguminosae	Samo
845. Woodsia mexicana Fée.	Polypodiaceae	
846. Xanthium canadense Mill.	Compositae	Cadio
847. Xanthium italicum Moretti in Tidest. & Kittell X. commune Britton	Compositae	Cadillos
848. Xanthium strumarium L. var. canadense (Mill.) Torr. & Gray	Compositae	Wisapole
849. Yucca baccata Torr. and Y. glauca Nutt. in Fras.	Liliaceae	Palmilla; Amole; Palmilla Ancha; Palma; Dátil; Yuca
850. Yucca decipiens Trel.	Liliaceae	Sotol; Palma de San Pedro; Palma; Palmilla

BOTANICAL NAME	FAMILY	SPANISH NAME
851. Yucca elata Engelm.	Liliaceae	Palmilla
852. Yucca glauca Nutt. in Fras. Y. angustifolia Pursh	Liliaceae	
853. Yucca sp.	Liliaceae	Amole; Flor de Palma; Yuca
854. Zaluzania triloba (Ort.) Pers.	Compositae	Alta Misa
855. Zea mays L.	Gramineae	Maiz; Flor de Maiz
856. Zexmenia podocephala	Compositae	Pionía;Peonía
857. Zingiber officinale Roscoe	Zingiberaceae	Ajenjibre
858. Zinnia acerosa (DC.) A.Gray Z. pumila A. Gray	Compositae	Manzanilla del Campo
859. Zinnia grandiflora Nutt.	Compositae	Cinco Llagas
860. Zinnia linearis Benth.	Compositae	Yerba del Torro
861. Zizyphus acuminata Benth.	Rhamnaceae	Vinjora
862. Zornia diphylla (L.) Pers.	Leguminosae	Hierba de Vibora; Yerba de la Vibora

BIBLIOGRAPHY

Arnberger, Leslie P.
1962 Flowers of the Southwest Mountains. Southwestern Monuments Association, Globe, Arizona.

Beal, Mary
1943 Incense Bush. Desert Magazine 6(8): 103-05.

Bennett, Wendell C. and Robert M. Zingg
1935 The Tarahumara, an Indian Tribe of Northern Mexico. University of Chicago Press, Chicago.

Carter, George F.
1947 A California Account of Uses of Medical Herbs. Western Folklore 6(3): 199-203.

Chavez, Tibo J.
1972 New Mexican Folklore of the Rio Abajo. Bishop Printing Company. Portales, New Mexico.

Clark, Margaret
1959 Health in the Mexican-American Culture. University of California Press, Berkeley.

Correll, D.S. and M.C. Johnston
1970 Manual of the Vascular Plants of Texas. Texas Research Foundation, Renner, Texas.

Craighead, John J., Frank C, Craighead, and Ray J. Davis
1963 A Field Guide to Rocky Mountain Wildflowers. Peterson Field Guide Series, No. 146. Houghton Middlin Co., Boston.

Curtin, L.S.M.
1947 Healing Herbs of the Upper Rio Grande.Laboratory of Anthropology, Santa Fe.

Dodge, Natt N.
1963 100 Desert Wildflowers. Southwestern Monuments Association, Globe, Arizona.
1965 Flowers of the Southwest Deserts. Southwestern Monuments Association, Globe, Arizona.
1967 100 Roadside Wildflowers. Southwestern Monuments Association, Globe, Arizona.

Field, Henry
1953 Notes of Medicinal Plants Used in Tepotzlan, Morelos, Mexico. América Indígena 13(4): 291-300.

Ford, Karen Cowan
(1966)* Ethnobotanical field notes from northern New Mexico. Collected primarily in 1966, some in 1967-1973.

Ford, Karen Cowan and Richard I.
(1965) A collection of medicinal herbs from the market in Ciudad Juarez, Chihuahua, Mexico.

Ford, Richard I.
1968 An Ecological Analysis Involving the Population of San Juan Pueblo, New Mexico. Ph.D. dissertation, University of Michigan, Ann Arbor, Michigan.

Foster, George M.
1953 Relations Between Spanish and Spanish-American Folk Medicine. Journal of American Folklore 66: 201-218.

Gonzalez, Nancie L.
1969 The Spanish-Americans of New Mexico. University of New Mexico Press, Albuquerque.

Goss, Arthur
1903 Ash Analysis of Some New Mexico Plants. New Mexico College of Agriculture and Mechanic Arts. Agricultural Experiment Station, Bulletin 44, Mesilla Park, New Mexico.

Havard, Valery
1895 Food Plants of the North American Indians. Bulletin of the Torrey Botanical Club 23(2): 33-46.

Holden, W.C. et al.
1936 Studies of the Yaqui Indians of Sonora, Mexico. Texas Technological College Bulletin 12(1), Lubbock.

Hrdlička, A.
1904 Notes on the Indians of Sonora. American Anthropologist, n.s. 6: 71-84.

Jones, Volney
(1931) The Ethnobotany of the Isleta Indians. M.A. thesis. University of New Mexico, Albuquerque.
(1932) Ethnobotanical field notes on medicinal herbs from market in Juarez, Chihuahua, Mexico.

Kearney, Thomas H. and Robert H. Peebles
1964 Arizona Flora. University of California Press, Berkeley.

* All dates enclosed in parentheses indicate unpublished material.

Kelly, Isabel T.
1965 Folk Practices in North Mexico. Institute of Latin American Studies, University of Texas, Latin American Monographs 2, Austin.

Lange, C.H.
1959 Cochiti: A New Mexico Pueblo, Past and Present. University of Texas Press, Austin.

Lloyd, C.G.
1914 Anemopsis californica -- the Yerba Mansa of the Pacific Coast. The Gleaner 4: 148-49, 161-62.

Lumholtz, Carl
1912 New Trails in Mexico. Charles Scribners, New York.

Lundell, C.L. and Alfred F. Whiting
(1934) Ethnobotanical field notes from Nueva Léón, Coahuilla and San Luís Potosí, México, for the University of Michigan.

Madsen, Claudia
1965 A Study of Change in Mexican Folk Medicine. Tulane University, Middle American Research Institute Publication 25: 89-138, New Orleans.

Madsen, William
1961 Society and Health in the Lower Rio Grande Valley. The Hogg Foundation for Mental Health, Austin.

Marquez, Mary N. and Consuelo Pacheco
1964 Midwifery Lore in New Mexico. American Journal of Nursing 64(9): 81-84.

Martin, William C., Charles R. Hutchins, and Robert G. Woodmansee
1970 A Flora of the Sandia Mountains. Department of Biology, The University of New Mexico, Albuquerque.

Martinez, Maximino
1959 Las Plantas Medicinales de México. México.

Meigs, Peveril, III
1939 The Kiliwa Indians of Lower California. Ibero-Americana 15, Berkeley.

Owen, Roger C.
1963 The Use of Plants and Non-magical Techniques in Curing Illness Among the Paipai, Santa Catarina, Baja California, Mexico. América Indígena 23(4): 319-344.

Palmer, Edward
1878 Plants Used by the Indians of the U.S. American Naturalist 12(9): 593-606; 12(10): 646-655.

Patraw, Pauline M.
1959 Flowers of the Southwest Mesas. Southwestern Monuments Association, Globe, Arizona.

Pennington, Campbell
1963_a_ Medicinal Plants Utilized by the Tepehuán of Southern Chihuahua. América Indígena 23(1): 31-47.
1963_b_ The Tarahumar of Mexico. University of Utah Press, Salt Lake City.

Redfield, Robert
1928 Remedial Plants of Tepotzlan: A Mexican Folk Herbal. Journal of the Washington Academy of Sciences 18(8): 216-26.

Riley, C.V.
1889 A Lac Insect on the Creosote Bush. Insect Life 1(11): 344-45.

Riley, Carroll L. and Carmen Trujillo
(1956) Herb collection from north Mexico.

Robbins, W.W., J.P. Harrington, and Barbara Freire-Marreco
1916 Ethnobotany of the Tewa Indians. Bureau of American Ethnology, Bulletin 55, Washington.

Rose, J.N.
1899 Notes on Useful Plants of Mexico. Contributions from the U.S. National Herbarium 5(4), Washington.

Russell, F.
1908 The Pima Indians. Annual Report of the Bureau of American Ethnology 26: 3-390, Washington.

Ruxton, George F.
1847 Adventures in Mexico and the Rocky Mountains. John Murray, London.

Schulman, Sam and Anne M. Smith
(1962) Health and Disease in Northern New Mexico: A Research Report. (First Phase, 1959-1960, U.S. P.H.S. RG-5615). Institute of Behavioral Science. University of Colorado, Boulder.

Sergeant, S.S.
(n.d.) Unpublished manuscript on useful plants of Tesuque and Santa Clara Pueblos, in possession of Edward P. Dozier. Data collected in the 1930s.

Shreve, Forrest and Ira L. Wiggins
1964 Vegetation and Flora of the Sonoran Desert. Stanford University Press, Stanford.

Standley, Paul
1920-1926 Trees and Shrubs of Mexico. Contributions from the U.S. National Herbarium. Vol. 23: part 1 (1920), part 2(1922), part 3(1923), part 4 (1924), part 5(1926). Government Printing Office, Washington.

Swadesh, Frances L.
1971 Crossroads of Culture: A New Mexico Bibliography. Museum of New Mexico Press, Santa Fe.

Tidestrom, Ivar and Sister Teresita Kittell
1941 A Flora of Arizona and New Mexico. The Catholic University of America Press, Washington.

Van der Eerden, Sister Lucia
1948 Maternity Care in a Spanish-American Community of New Mexico. The Catholic University of America Anthropological Series 13, Washington.

White, Leslie
(1941) A collection of herbs from B. Ruppe's drugstore, Albuquerque, New Mexico.

Wooton, E.O.
1894 New Mexico Weeds. New Mexico College of Agriculture and the Mechanic Arts. Agricultural Experiment Station, Bulletin 13, Las Cruces.

Wooton, E.O. and Paul Standley
1915 Flora of New Mexico. Contributions from the U.S. National Herbarium 19, Washington.

Zingg, Robert M.
1932 Mexican Folk Remedies of Chihuahua. Journal of the Washington Academy of Sciences 22(7): 174-181.

www.ingramcontent.com/pod-product-compliance
Lightning Source LLC
Jackson TN
JSHW070312120426
100741JS00007B/32

* 9 7 8 0 9 3 2 2 0 6 5 8 9 *